BY JORGE CRUISE

THE
CRUISE CONTROL™
DIET

THE
CRUISE C⏱NTROL™
DIET

AUTOMATE YOUR DIET AND CONQUER WEIGHT LOSS FOREVER

JORGE CRUISE

BALLANTINE BOOKS
NEW YORK

Copyright © 2019 by Jorge Cruise Media, Inc.

Published in the United States by Ballantine Books, an imprint of Random House, a division of Penguin Random House LLC, New York.

BALLANTINE and the HOUSE colophon are registered trademarks of Penguin Random House LLC.

Hardback ISBN 9780525618690
Ebook ISBN 9780525618706

Printed in the United States of America on acid-free paper

randomhousebooks.com

9 8 7 6 5 4 3 2 1

First Edition

Book design by Diane Hobbing

To Sam

CONTENTS

FOREWORD

Brooke Burke, CEO and founder of Brooke Burke Body and CEO of Modern Mom

"Pass the butter, please." The barista at Starbucks gave me a crazy look. My bestie Jorge and I exchanged *that* smile, the one that says, "If you only knew, you'd be buttering up all the coffee."

At first, it might be shocking. Jorge is bringing a message that encourages us to do many of the things we've been trained *not* to do. Here's the thing. I always say that I'm Jorge's physical "Body of Evidence," because I've been consistently following Cruise Control for the past two years and I've never had such high energy, health, and mood and such low body fat in my life. It's not about the weight really because I'm not a girl who's paying attention to the numbers on a scale. It's an optimal eating style that allows you to enjoy life along the way. Jorge is the king of simplifying healthy lifestyles. This plan is fun, comprehensive, and it really works. I'm a fitness and wellness junkie with four children and too many jobs, and I'm in the best shape of my life at forty-seven years old thanks to Cruise Control! *And,* it's automatic. I don't have to think about it. You can trust Jorge and the Cruise Control method for a successful way to change your relationship with food, blast fat, and enjoy every delicious bite of it along the way. This life trajectory is a simple health course that will change your life.

The bottom line is, Jorge's philosophies work and he walks his talk—with a backpack full of unexpected goodies. He usually comes along packing high-fat natural goodies, a grinder full of Himalayan pink salt, and carrying two plates full of food to show you how you can eat more, burn fat, and lose weight.

Take this opportunity to reset your lifestyle with the least amount of effort. Don't take my word for it. See me as a body of evidence, and Jorge as your guide to share a new philosophy, at a brand-new speed.

Cruise Control is getting from point A to point B in the quickest amount of time. It's about finding the right pace and comfort zone to fit your unique journey. It's an age-old secret made new. It works, and now it's yours.

INTRODUCTION

Dr. Jason Fung

There are thousands of diet books on the market, and I think I must have read them all: low-fat diets, low-carb diets, low-calorie diets, paleo diets, keto diets. All of these diets work if you follow them carefully . . . at least at first. The pounds fly off. Everything goes exactly as advertised. Life is sweet. But this honeymoon period usually only lasts for about six months.

Then, slowly, almost imperceptibly, the diet's power seems to wane. The pounds are not flying off, but the scale is still moving in the right direction, just a little slower. Then slower. Then slower again. So, you redouble your efforts. You go lower fat, or lower carb, or lower calorie than ever. This intensified effort pays dividends, but not at the rate of weight loss you enjoyed at the start.

Then the dreaded, inevitable day comes, as you always knew it would. The pounds stop coming off completely—a plateau. But it's still all good, you tell yourself. As long as the weight stays at this level, you'll be happy. But your happiness is short-lived. Because despite your maximum efforts, your weight starts to budge upward. Slowly at first. But with growing horror, you see it accelerate. Within a year, or two at the maximum, your weight is back where it was when all this effort to lose weight began. You are crushed. You are devastated. You know you've tried your best, even as you face the silent accusations and crushing condescension of your friends and family. Again.

It happens to the best of us. If you've ever watched any of the weight-loss competition shows on television, you'll know that insane amounts of exercise combined with highly restricted diets can produce very impressive results, but only in the short term. You might have noticed that they never have reunion shows because all the contestants have gained their weight back. In many cases, their weight is higher than before they started the show!

Why? Why do so many of us struggle with losing weight—and keeping it off? I've spent my career studying this problem and discovering the solution.

I trained at the University of Toronto and the University of California, Los Angeles, to become a doctor and kidney specialist. But after years in practice, I realized that many metabolic diseases, such as obesity and type 2 diabetes, must be treated with diet, not medications. I, along with most other doctors, had missed the seemingly self-evident point that dietary diseases must be treated with diet, not drugs. Now we see it: using medications for a dietary problem was as useful as bringing a snorkel to a bicycle race.

Today, I run an Intensive Dietary Management (IDM) clinic in Toronto, where I've been seeing patients for eighteen years. I've been in the daily fight to help people lose weight and keep it off, and I've been researching and writing about weight loss for ten years, too.

Both in my clinic and in polite company, everyone asks the same question: What should I eat? What's the magic combination of ingredients and quantities? Should we eat avocados or kale? Should we eat bacon or skinless turkey breast? Should I eat vegetables or meat?

But here's what all of my thought and experience tells me: what to eat is only half the equation.

Questions about diet—ingredient questions—don't get at the other key part of the equation: timing questions. They fail to address whether we should eat three meals or six, early in the day or later at night. In fact, most diets completely ignore this "when" question altogether. It's therefore no wonder they've all failed to deliver the promised weight benefits over the long term. No matter how much we adjust the foods we eat, if we don't acknowledge and change the timing of our eating, we won't be successful. We can change what we eat and we can eat healthier ingredients—quinoa, cabbage soup, leafy greens. But that's only half the problem. And you can't ignore half the problem and expect great results. After all, if you answer half the questions on the final exam, the highest mark you can get is an F.

Think back to the 1970s, before the obesity epidemic. Take a look at an old photograph from that era, perhaps a street scene. What is incredible is just how little obesity there is. Take a look at some old high school yearbooks from the 1970s. There is virtually no obesity. Perhaps one child in a hundred.

What was the diet of the 1970s? They were eating white bread and jam. They were eating ice cream. They were eating Oreo cookies. They were not eating whole-wheat pasta. They were not eating quinoa. They were not eating kale. They were not counting calories. They were not counting net carbs. They were not even really exercising much. These people were doing everything "wrong," yet seemingly effortlessly there was no obesity. Why? The answer is simple. Come closer. Listen carefully.

They were not eating all the time.

That's all. Large-scale surveys from 1977 showed that most Americans ate three times per day. Breakfast, lunch, and dinner. If you wanted an after-school snack, your mom said, "No, you'll ruin your dinner." If you wanted a bedtime snack, your mom said, "You should have eaten more at dinner." By contrast, the average person today eats six or more times per day over about fifteen hours. Think about this in real terms: this means that the average person eats breakfast at 8:00 A.M. and doesn't stop eating until 10:45 P.M.! The only time we are not eating is when we are sleeping. Grazing is great . . . if you are a cow or want to look like one.

The physiology of weight gain is not very complicated. Your body really only exists in two states—the fed state and the fasted state. When you eat (fed state), insulin goes up, which signals the body to store some of this incoming food energy as body fat. When you don't eat (fasted state), insulin levels fall, and this signals the body to use some of this stored food energy. We need this to feed our brain, our heart, our lungs, our kidneys, and so on. Your body can either store fat or burn fat, but not both at the same time.

If we spend our entire day in the fed state, then we are constantly storing fat. In the 1970s, if you ate breakfast at 8:00 A.M. and dinner at 6:00 P.M., then you spent ten hours of the day in the fed state (storing fat) and fourteen hours of the day in the fasted state (burning fat). This balance between storing fat and burning fat kept obesity rates low. Today we spend almost fifteen hours a day storing fat, and only nine hours a day burning it. It doesn't take a genius to figure out why body fat increases!

I've taken this realization to heart in my IDM clinic. I have asked patients to change their diet, but also to add in periods of fasting. And I've written about my methods in two books, *The Obesity Code* and *The Complete Guide to Fasting*. The results I saw—some of which I have shared in my books—were almost unbelievable. Patients were losing hundreds of pounds, seemingly effortlessly. Patients were coming off the diabetic medications. It was incredible. The best part was that we were improving people's health, giving them back control over their own body using a technique that was free, available, and used for millennia by virtually every civilization in the history of the world!

Now Jorge Cruise takes the next leap forward, making this ageless wisdom easier to apply to your everyday life. One innovative feature is his use of healthy fats to make fasting easier. Pure dietary fat has almost no effect on the fat-storing hormone insulin, so it offers a simple hack to kill hunger pangs while allowing all the benefits of fasting. Genius. By setting out a simple fasting schedule, Jorge allows you to set yourself on Cruise Control for an automated journey back to health and wellness.

Jason Fung, M.D.
Author, *The Obesity Code* and *The Complete Guide to Fasting*

WELCOME!

This book presents information and a plan that will change your life. I know this because it changed mine, too.

Three years ago, I had a picture-perfect life—a fantastic marriage, two wonderful sons, and a jet-setting lifestyle as a celebrity trainer. My days were packed with work to build my brand—writing blogs, articles, and recipes; jumping from meetings to press appearances; and working with clients—online and in person. I was also in the middle of launching a new podcast with actress and host Brooke Burke and developing a new workout method. Oh, and I lived in sunny, happy, shiny Malibu—things were great indeed!

But I was just so tired from burning the candle at both ends. On the rare occasions that I did have time off, I was irritable, unable to relax, and couldn't enjoy my time with the people I love most. Despite feeling completely shattered and ready to hit my pillow every night, I was always too mentally wound up and couldn't fall asleep, so I'd get up and stretch or meditate or breathe slowly or tense and relax my muscles or visualize counting sheep. Or all of those things! You name it, I tried it. But I just couldn't relax. I'd end up getting five to six hours of tossing and turning "sleep" a night, and I'd wake up just as fried as I'd felt the night before—only to start the whole cycle over again.

And sleep wasn't my only problem. I also felt as though no matter how much I exercised, I was struggling to maintain a healthy weight, and I wasn't in peak fitness. What I had always done (cardio in the morning and weight training in the evening) wasn't giving me the same kind of lean and toned-up results I used to get. Indeed, I was having to work out harder and longer to keep up my physique, but it wasn't working. I'm not sure that anyone would have noticed that I wasn't quite as hard-bodied as I once was, but *I knew*.

And given that I make my living helping others look and feel good— and that the *New York Times* once dubbed me a "suntanned fitness guru"—it was essential that I do something to turn this strange situation around. I really needed to look and feel my best. Don't we all?

Now, I've written a lot of books about how to fuel and move your body for optimal results. I know that what you put in your mouth is 80 percent of the issue for most people. Exercise definitely matters, but eating a low-carb, high-fat, and moderate-protein diet is generally the best way to burn belly fat, lose weight, and gain fitness. Based on these tenets, my bestselling books—including *8 Minutes in the Morning,* the Belly Fat series, and, more recently, *The 100*—have helped millions of people lose weight and keep it off. My readers and clients write to me all the time to tell me that they love my programs, recipes, and meal planners, and my iPhone and Facebook page are full of photos of clients that show the great results in weight loss and fat burning, and gains in fitness, health, and happiness that people report. What I'm saying is, I was in a great position to figure out the source of my problem!

MY JOURNEY TO CRUISE CONTROL

So, I scrutinized my diet. Was I eating in a way that was somehow counterproductive? At the time, my daily intake looked something like this: I had three low-carb and good meals a day—I'd start with a power breakfast (usually oatmeal and a protein shake), and I didn't eat junk or processed foods at lunch or dinner, either. To boot, I always had a healthy snack before *and* after my workouts (a banana before and a protein bar or nuts afterward). I ate clean, lean, and often to fuel my workouts and keep my energy high.

I was doing everything right! I clearly needed to call in reinforcements!

Here's another thing that's wonderful about my life: my position gives me access to the best scientific minds in the fitness and nutrition realms. If I have a question or a concern, I can call the lab scientists and academic experts who are doing cutting-edge work on metabolism or energy or cell regeneration. So I called. I talked to Dr. Satchin Panda, of the Salk Institute and author of *The Circadian Code.* I picked Mark Sisson's brain. Sisson is a triathlete and author of *The Primal Blueprint.* I consulted with Dr. Catherine Shanahan, creator of the L.A. Lakers PRO Nutrition Program and author of *Deep Nutrition*. And I quizzed Dr. Jason Fung, founder of the Intensive Dietary Management Program and author of *The Complete Guide to Fasting*. These people are on the front, front lines. They—or the people they work with—publish hundreds of papers every year and their contributions are constantly informing my recommendations for tweaks to make to our diets here and there.

What all these luminaries—and many more—agreed on was that science was starting to understand and prove the power of a term Dr. Fung had in his book title: *intermittent fasting*. For you and me, think of it as *the power of when*.

Or, as Dr. Panda and his colleagues put it: *"When we eat is as important as what we eat."* They first stumbled upon this stunning breakthrough in animal studies. When they gave mice the run of the house during a set period of time, the mice lost weight. When they put mice on a restricted diet and fed them throughout the day, they gained weight. Their amazing conclusion: by limiting the period of time in which you're consuming food, you actually increase the number of calories—especially fat calories—your body burns during the day.

More specifically, *the science was proving that an eight-hour time-restricted eating window and a sixteen-hour fasting window was the magic formula*.

We'll get into this in more detail in Chapter 1, but here's the short version: Intermittent fasting (having a regular period of not eating for at least sixteen hours a day) signals your body to burn fat while speeding up your muscle growth and accelerating your metabolism—automatically. Intermittent fasting for just part of your day signals your body's repair systems to replace used-up and worn-out cells. These cellular mechanics can't work on your brain and body if you eat all the time.

I had an aha moment: My wake-to-sleep eating habits were one of the main reasons I was feeling so lousy. I was blocking my body from crucial functions by my lack of *not-eating* time.

A second aha. By including a period of *not eating* (intermittent fasting), I could call in the cellular repair crew and turn on some remarkably magical abilities that would trigger effortless weight loss, fat burning, increased energy, better sleep, lower stress, and a happier life.

I have to be honest: the more I learned, the more this breakthrough got me really excited. My husband, Sam, would tell you that I was zipping around like my younger son after he's scarfed down a package of Sour Patch Kids. Yes, I was fired up! Because the science also showed that the eight hours of time-restricted eating (TRE) and sixteen hours of intermittent fasting were not only great for weight loss, muscle tone, and more energy! Intermittent fasting was also proving to be the secret sauce to reducing inflammation throughout the body, which in turn reduces risks for all kinds of nasty and life-threatening diseases and symptoms—and increases your life span.

In addition to all that, because this technique is not about *what* you are eating, it will work regardless of which eating style you follow. From keto to vegan—you can use intermittent fasting to speed up your body's ability to burn fat, to lose weight, and to improve health—because you're paying attention to *when* first and foremost. Furthermore, paying attention to *when* you eat doesn't require any of us to restrict food groups, count points, track calories, or exercise for hours and hours. In other words, when you focus on when, you can *automate* your eating—you don't have to think about all those other criteria.

Sounds great, right? But wait, you say! If this were a TV sitcom, we'd all be hearing that screeching brake effect. As in, "Wait a minute! Did you say fasting? For sixteen hours? Jorge, what the what?"

MY FIRST ATTEMPTS AT INTERMITTENT FASTING

I'm with you: the word "fasting" freaked me out, too. It made me think of a gaunt, skeletal guy in a robe meditating up on some desert mountain—*not* my idea of a good time. Besides, the way I'd been working out, I assumed that having healthy munchies within arm's reach at all times was a necessity, not overkill. I wasn't about to start telling my clients and fans that they should be doing something that sounded kind of extreme.

But I *was* willing to start experimenting on myself (you're welcome)!

The first thing I thought was: Hey, you're already technically fasting overnight (a.k.a. sleeping). So, right there that's eight hours. I just needed to extend my intermittent fasting period another eight hours. I did that by skipping breakfast and got rid of the little bags of snacks I had always relied on to "fuel" me all day long. I held out to have a big afternoon lunch. With an eight-hour window to eat, I was able to have a nice dinner at a more or less regular time.

I also worked on some new terminology, because try as I might to embrace intermittent fasting as a concept, I kept thinking of that emaciated guy on a mountaintop. My solution, instead of thinking in terms of intermittent fasting and time-restricted eating cycles (the eating portion of intermittent fasting), was to think in terms of "burning" (since the fasting part of intermittent fasting triggers your body's fat-*burning* engine) and "boosting" (since the eating portion usually *boosts* your energy). Hence, the use of the phrases "Burn Zone" and "Boost Zone," which you'll learn much more about in a few pages (or you can jump ahead to page 26 for details). Words are powerful to the mind! My use of those phrases may sound trivial, but they take out the negative feeling of deprivation that comes from the word "fasting" and the highly regimented feeling from the word "restricted." Both of these words focus on what you can't do, while *burning* and *boosting* focus on what you, your brain, and your body can do.

And you know what happened? I lost seven pounds after the first seven days of Boosting and Burning! I lost that weight and kept it off, effortlessly. I noticed the return of a younger self's stamina and energy. I felt like my body and brain had found some new sort of super-fuel. I was stunned. I just thought this new plan might help me relax and enjoy life a little more, but I had no idea it would prove to be a weight-loss, energy-revving, and fat-burning miracle.

MY INTERMITTENT INNOVATION

All that said, I discovered—not too surprisingly—that not eating for sixteen hours was hard! I have to admit it: I was hungry a lot. And toward the end of the sixteen-hour period? I was also tired—my energy levels definitely dipped.

But see, I loved the results of intermittent fasting (a.k.a. Burning). I was hooked on this new idea, and I was just as determined to come up with a solution that wouldn't compromise the benefits of a sixteen-hour intermittent fast but would make it easier.

Drumroll, please. Lucky for you (and me, too!), I have found a scientific loophole that demolishes hunger pangs and keeps energy revved up.

This is my innovation: *You're going to cheat your fast with fat!*

Car brake screech again. Am I right? How can I tell you that you can fast *and* eat simultaneously?

Back to the science: it turns out that certain healthy fats don't disrupt your body's fasting state. Meaning, you can enjoy certain treats during your sixteen-hour intermittent fast as a way to combat hunger and cravings, but your body won't "know" it. With healthy fats, you can still physically stay in an intermittently fasted state that boosts weight loss, fat burning, and also energy and mood, without any of the hunger pangs and food cravings that make hours of abstinence such a bitch (excuse my French). You'll learn all about these foods, when and how to use them and why they work, in the chapters that follow. For now, just know that they make fasting effortless. And know that we're going to call them Burn Zone beverages and treats (this is how you'll get all the benefits of intermittent fasting with none of the downsides).

I call my technique Cruise Control not just because my last name is Cruise, but also because it is a method that is so effortless, it quickly becomes automatic. It gives your body what it needs to perform well, tells your brain that all is well, and provides all the metabolic benefits of a fast. If you want to shed fat and improve your health as quickly and effortlessly as possible, you'll find it hard to beat Cruise Control.

My Cruise Control technique also works better because it increases how protein is processed in your body to help you to build muscle better. And it turns out that when you incorporate healthy fats into your mornings, you help your body to switch into fat-burning mode faster, even if you had carbohydrates the day before.

Cruise Control is a paradigm shift. This plan eliminates willpower. It eliminates sacrifice. And it eliminates calorie counting, glycemic-index crunching, carb-fat-protein balancing, point totaling, and other Einsteinian math-nastics that have turned ordering dinner into an arithmetic problem worthy of Harvard Business School. Instead, just eat the foods you love, but focus on when to eat each day.

When you start focusing not on the number of calories you consume but rather on when to eat, your body will respond in kind, revving up its fat burning and nutrient absorption and naturally regulating your caloric intake. This results in the weight loss and mental clarity that so many people are already experiencing on Cruise Control. I know my program works— I've tested it on myself and on countless clients.

Are you game? I hope so! You're going to see amazing benefits. I know that you can lose as much as twenty-eight pounds in as many days on this plan; the more you have to lose, the faster the weight will come off to start.

When I met Oprah Winfrey for the first time more than twenty years ago, she told me, "The key to helping the most amount of people is to keep things simple." That's something I've always tried to do, and this book is the ultimate program in print that will put you in the driver's seat to your simplest and best life ever. So, take a breath—now take another one—now, open your mind and join me on the road to understanding that *timing is everything*!

THE
CRUISE CONTROL™
DIET

CHAPTER 1

Timing Is Everything

Do the best you can until you know better. Then when you know better, do better.

—MAYA ANGELOU

hat's the best way to lose weight and improve your health? For years you've been promised countless, clashing, opposing, and misleading "best" practices for the *one* way to lose weight successfully. Let's take a look at just some of these:

- You must count calories.
- You shouldn't count calories.
- Don't eat fat; fat makes you fat.
- Do eat fat; carbs make you fat.
- You should eat fresh fruits and vegetables.
- You shouldn't eat any fruit.
- You can eat as much fruit as you want.

- Eat only sugar, only on special occasions or on weekends, while standing on one foot.
- Just eat what our ancestors ate.
- It's impossible to eat paleo.
- Count points, not calories.
- Count only your carbs.
- Count only sugar calories.
- Eat frequently.
- Eat only three times a day; never skip breakfast.
- Cardio burns fat best.
- Strength training revs your metabolism.

And on and on it goes!

Regardless of how absurd or conflicting, every diet plan can basically be divided into one of two groups.

Calorie-Restrictive Diets: These weight-loss strategies all include methods for eating fewer calories than your body requires—creating a calorie debt. Here are the kitchens equipped with food scales and measuring cups and spoons; and pantries, cupboards, and fridges packed with low-cal and low-fat foods that include rice cakes, fat-free cottage cheese, and water-packed tuna—don't forget the melba toast, lettuce, and grapefruit. Most of these calorie-counting diets also coincided with the low-fat frenzy that began to be popular in the 1970s and '80s. The logic used here was that as long as you eat fewer calories than your body burns each day, you'll lose weight. It's a great idea, but . . .

The problem with this logic is that calorie counting is an overly simplistic way of viewing nutrition and how the human body is biologically designed; it assumes that your stomach is like a simple furnace that burns up the food you eat in a very 2 + 2 = 4 sort of way. If this was the way our bodies functioned, we'd all be able to subject our diets to some basic math, and voilà, we'd be slim and sleek. Not exactly, right? Because our bodies don't work like that. We are far more complex. Your body takes the food you put in your mouth and breaks it down into components (a.k.a. macronutrients) that you eat, and then uses these nutrients for different purposes—to build muscle, to run marathons, to yell at the kids (or husband) to pick up their socks! Some of these reactions inside your body cause fat burning, while others cause the accumulation of fat.

Calorie-restrictive diets are based on deprivation and restriction, and they increasingly bash your willpower and slow your metabolism, until you find yourself in a blackout with a container of cookie dough in your hand with no memory of how it got there. It's a one-two punch that doesn't fool your body for a second. Your body knows when it's being deprived, and it sends out alert signals (powerful ones), and the result, sooner or later, is you off your diet feeling like a miserable failure. It's not your fault.

What's worse is that when you finally do give in (and you will) and have a day of eating that includes even a "normal" amount, your body greedily gobbles it all up and stores the food as fat in your body. It's a sensible reaction if you think about it from your poor starving body's point of view: "Hey, this jerk has decided to let us eat today. Let's save as much as we can for the next time he tries to take away our food!" The result: you gain more weight than you lost.

Hormones become imbalanced and your body panics and stores fat. You feel constantly hungry, foggy, and unfocused, and you'll be tired all the time. Oh, and it won't work. This is the main reason that we're living the blob-ish existence that life has become, but it doesn't have to be like this.

After many years of trying in vain to cut calories to lose weight, a new strategy started to surface. The Atkins diet, South Beach, the Wheat Belly Diet, and many other food plans that focused on restricting certain foods began to trend in the 1990s and later. Unfortunately, these diets come with their own challenges.

Food-Restrictive Diets: These are what I consider the "new-school" way of losing weight. Eat all you want, just don't eat any carbs, or wheat, or fat, or fruit, or meat, or dairy, or sugar, or anything else you might remotely enjoy. Or foods that paleo men didn't eat. Or foods that aren't raw.

Restricting whole food groups goes against your biology. Our bodies are made to eat and process carbohydrates, fats, *and* proteins. Each macronutrient provides a different service and gives your body the nutrients you require for optimal functioning. Unless you have a severe allergy to a certain food (for instance, peanuts, milk, or strawberries), there is no sane reason to completely banish any natural, unprocessed, or whole food from your shopping list. And you definitely don't want to cut out an entire category.

Food-restrictive diets are just too limiting. If you've tried one, you know what I'm talking about! Cutting out whole food groups or avoiding entire sections of your supermarket is an exercise in denying your uniqueness—one person might love eating only protein and greens, while another responds to a no-bread rule like a two-pack-a-day smoker who's been cut off cold turkey. In other words, food restriction messes with your mind. You tell yourself you absolutely can't have chocolate cake. What happens? You suddenly *must* have chocolate cake. It's all you can think about. It's like saying, "No matter what, don't think of a pink elephant"—suddenly, your imagination is flooded with a herd of blushing beasts.

Of course, some diets blend both strategies—requiring you to dramatically cut calories *and* food groups, which ends up being even less fun, and more ineffective. The truth is that any and all of these methods will work for most people for a short time because if you dramatically change the amount or kind of food you eat, your body will react by shedding some weight. But will those changes last? If you're reading this book, you know. And you may have also discovered another uncomfortable truth: sometimes losing weight through a dramatic change in your diet results in weight *gain*!

As much as you might want to blame yourself for your weight and health problems, I'm here to tell you that it isn't your fault. As evidenced by the list at the beginning of this chapter, you've been fed a lot of nonsense or downright bad advice, and you are not alone.

Plus, consider the fact that we have become a culture of grazing beings. Snacking as an American pastime has reached an all-time high—today nibbling and noshing outside of our three main meals is something around 95 percent of us do at least once a day, while more than 60 percent of us regularly eat four or more snacks each day. Why? It's what you've been taught. Your doctor may have even told you that it's healthier to eat frequently all day long. You've read, heard, or been straight-out told that snacking will keep your blood sugar from getting too low, will help rev up your calorie-burning engine, will keep you from ever feeling hungry (God forbid), will stop your bingeing, will better provide you with all the nutrients you need, et cetera. Wake up! You're about to learn that none of these things are true—it's actually *this* constant noshing that is the main reason obesity rates and diseases related to obesity continue to increase.

THE FAST TRACK TO AUTOMATIC HEALTH

Continuous eating is like overusing your car. If you overuse an engine and never let it cool down, you'll burn it out and end up with a hunk of metal that no longer works. The same holds true for your body. If you are always eating, you repeatedly trigger your body to produce certain chemicals—especially the one that regulates fat making and fat storing: insulin. Frequent feeding compromises your body's ability to properly regulate the energy you take in and leads to weight gain and excess fat.

Think about the family car you had when you were growing up. Ours was a beige 1980-something Ford truck—standard transmission. It overheated—a lot—and there was no automatic anything: no air-conditioning, no power steering, no automatic windows, and definitely no cruise control. Today's cars can run on electricity, they have automatic everything—remote start-ups, windows, doors, lock, unlock, and, of course, you can put them on autopilot. Today I drive a 2017 Porsche Macan SUV. I drive a lot, from Malibu to San Diego (and if you're from Southern California, you know that L.A. traffic is *the* worst), so I wanted to invest in a car that would comfortably hold me as well as my family. Some weeks I drive so much that my car can feel like a second home. The ride is as smooth and quiet as silk. Everything operates at the touch of a button. The soft leather seats are kid-friendly, and with fourteen-way adjustable controls, the seats are the most comfortable I've ever been in. Did I mention that the seats are air-conditioned and heated? It's impossible to leave keys in the car or any of the doors open—there are alerts for everything. Of course, we have cruise control, but not just the run-of-the-mill set-the-speed-and-go-auto-pilot cruising. We are talking *adaptive* cruise control. That means that you tell your car how far you want to stay ahead of and behind the cars around you and it slows, accelerates, stops, and reaccelerates all without you touching the gas or brake pedal.

I could go on and on—it's all pretty cool—but even with all the bells and whistles, a car is still a car. Four wheels that take you from point A to B. But you can either get there in an uncomfortable, hot/cold, and unreliable vehicle, or you can get there in style! And isn't that what you want with your weight loss? To get to your "destination" in as much comfort as possible? That's what the Cruise Control plan is all about. You'll get to forever weight loss, fat burning, and you'll be healthier and happier, but you are going to enjoy the "ride" a whole lot more. On Cruise Control, your body will know how to speed up, slow down, and stop, all without your having to be mentally and physically tied to the mechanics of driving. You're about to experience a new and improved way to reach your goals—and you'll get better mileage *and* performance out of your "machine" to boot.

WHAT MAKES YOU FAT & UNHEALTHY

Before we jump into the automating-your-weight-loss part, a little biology lesson is required. When you understand why you are overweight in the first place, you'll be able to clearly see how and why Cruise Control is going to work—forever.

Insulin is the hormone that makes you fat. Did you get that? It's not too much food, it's insulin—*not* excess calories. Insulin is like the Hulk when it comes to getting fat. I know the Hulk can be a good guy, but he can also wreak a lot of havoc and blow up if he gets angry. Well, insulin is like that—it can be good, and even as mellow as Bruce Banner, but if you bombard insulin with too many of the wrong foods, *at the wrong times*—look out!

Insulin's main purpose is to store fat (energy) to protect you from starving. In the past, when we were hunter-gatherer nomad types, this came in handy. There wasn't always food available, and we needed our fat stores to give us energy to get us through the tough times when food was scarce. Today, most of us can and do get food whenever we desire. We can drive through, order delivery, pick up, take out—or just open the fridge—day or night. But your body doesn't understand the difference, which is why we still produce insulin and store fat as though we were cavemen!

Of course, there are many other hormones and body chemicals that are involved with hunger, appetite, cravings, feeling full, and other nuances of storing fat, but insulin is the star—the Big Enchilada that tells your body what to do with the food you eat. One of insulin's main jobs is to move glucose (your blood sugar) from your bloodstream into your cells so that it can be used for energy. Here's the way it is supposed to work: You eat something; the food you eat spikes your blood sugar; this spike triggers a signal to your pancreas telling it to produce and release insulin. Now, with insulin as the escort, your cells will let the glucose come inside to be used or stored as energy. This is why you often hear of insulin being described as a key because glucose can't *open the door* without the key (a.k.a. insulin) to get from your bloodstream to inside your cell. The problem we have today—an epidemic of obesity, metabolic disease, and diabetes—is that we are eating too much, too often, and the foods we are choosing spike insulin. This is what makes you fat.

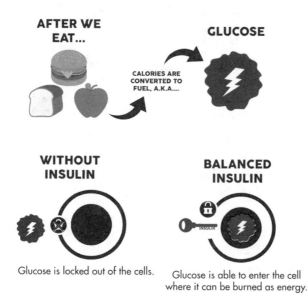

AFTER WE EAT...

GLUCOSE

CALORIES ARE CONVERTED TO FUEL, A.K.A....

WITHOUT INSULIN

BALANCED INSULIN

Glucose is locked out of the cells.

Glucose is able to enter the cell where it can be burned as energy.

You may have heard of insulin in a slightly different context: insulin resistance. More than eighty-four million Americans are now at risk of being insulin resistant—that's about one out of three adults in the United States. But what does it mean?

If you have insulin resistance, it means that the receptors on the membranes of the cells (the locks) that are made to work with insulin (the key) don't respond like they are supposed to—they are no longer sensitive to insulin. This leads to a buildup of glucose in the blood.

The pancreas responds to foods that chronically spike insulin by going into overproduction mode. Your pancreas tries to produce extra insulin to force glucose into your cells. However, your body "reads" all this excess insulin as an alarm to store the food away as fat, and not to burn up the calories you eat. This is why you get fat.

INSULIN RESISTANCE

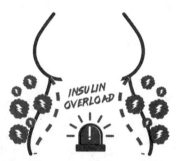

In response, your pancreas produces more and more insulin, which signals the body to store the excess glucose as fat.

If only we could text our body the way that we can instantly message our friends, and tell it not to store food as fat. Unfortunately, that's not how it works. And it shows. The way we eat today has more than 75 percent of us struggling with overweight and obesity, and usually that comes with related conditions such as diabetes, heart disease, high blood pressure, cancer, and more. Just look around. If you're not battling any extra pounds yourself, you know someone who is—I'd bet my Porsche Macan on it! We've turned insulin into a green beast with our modern-day eating habits, food choices, and constant availability of food.

But here's the thing: even though you can't send your body an instant message, you *can* tell it to *stop* the fat-storing madness.

THE POWER OF THE CLOCK

The way you stop the clock on storing fat is to start respecting the many timing systems that help your body run, well, like clockwork.

You already know that cutting out calories or banishing categories of food won't work. The most effective way to lower your insulin levels is to pay attention to *when* you eat. That's right, the timing of eating is the piece we've been missing.

Yes, the quality of what you eat is important—and as you'll see, my diet pays close attention to the optimal combination of fat, protein, and carbohydrates—but, let me repeat, the real power to effortless weight loss and fat burning is in the timing.

Your body runs on a timing system, and not just one. Scientists call these clocks circadian rhythms. You have a master clock in your brain, but you also have clocks in your gut, your eyes, your pancreas, and more. In fact, it turns out that you have clocks in just about every cell in your body. You have a clock in your stomach that tells you when to be hungry and when to be full, a clock in your brain that tells you when to get sleepy and when to wake up, another that tells you when to have a bowel movement, and so on. The problem is that our clocks don't do so well in conjunction with our modern lifestyles—we've knocked our timing systems all out of whack. What we are missing is synchronicity.

Think back again to early humans. Once upon a time, we lived according to the natural rhythms of the day: sunrise and sunset, the seasons of the year, and the weather of each day. We woke and slept according to dawn and dusk, and we ate according to what we could gather or hunt. During the winter, when days were shorter, darker, and colder, we ate less and slept more. Vice versa in the summer. All of our clocks used to line up. We got hungry when we were naturally awake, and food was available, and we stopped eating and slept when the sun went down. We had to be fully active during the day and physically interactive with all parts of living—hunting and gathering, building shelter, finding water, making clothing—nothing was automated. Today we are about as far from those Paleolithic times as possible—we are awake before it gets light and we stay awake long after it gets dark. We no longer need to physically exert ourselves to get food, build shelter, or make clothes. Thanks to Amazon and Blue Apron, you don't even have to leave your house to get groceries, toiletries, or clothing. Food is available 24/7, exercise is something you need a gym membership for, and sleeping has become something you might pop a pill to experience.

I'm simplifying here, but it's easy to see that we no longer flow with our natural rhythms, the way we were designed to exist, and it's thrown our timing off. The results are brains that no longer know when to get sleepy, stomachs that no longer know natural hunger or satisfaction, and bodies that don't get the activity they need.

GRETCHEN THE GRAZER—A TRUE CLIENT STORY

I used to work with an actress I'll call Gretchen. At the time, she was in production on a TV show and had to be available for scenes until around 1:00 P.M. She would wake up and start her day with a heavy protein shake with peanut butter, honey, protein powder, and milk. Gretchen and I usually met at around 1:00 P.M., and before we'd work out she'd have another protein shake, this time with a banana. Then we'd do an interval workout, and she'd finish with a three-mile run. At the end of the workout, yep, she'd have yet another protein shake. This time she'd have it with a chicken salad or a veggie wrap that she believed she needed in addition to the shake because of all the calories she just got done burning. For dinner, Gretchen would have her final protein shake of the day with another salad or some sort of grilled chicken and veggies. Our training sessions were intense, around two hours a day, but then she was eating all day long. The ingredients were healthy overall, but she was eating too much, too often, and for too long of a time span over the day. The result was that Gretchen was constantly battling weight fluctuations. Her main problem was that she never let her body get hungry.

You and your body need to get hungry. Your body can only complete certain critical tasks when you allow a period of time when you don't eat. The research shows that when you eat throughout the day, your body is more likely to store fat and gain weight, while other areas of your body (the ones that rely on not eating) can't perform specific essential functions in your body if you are always eating. In fact, when you eat all the time, your body can't rest, replenish, and restore cells all over your body and in your brain—and the result is the epidemic of overweight, obesity, diabetes, heart disease, cancer, insomnia, stress, anxiety, and depression we see in our world.

THE ANCIENT SECRET OF HEALTH—FASTING!

So, the power of eating less frequently sends the *message* to your body to produce less insulin and store less fat. This brings us to a powerful and doable conclusion: the answer to your dieting woes is to create recurrent and long-enough periods of not eating (fasting) so that your body can stop storing fat and start burning it.

Again, research bears this out: When researchers from the Salk Institute, led by Dr. Satchin Panda, had people restrict their eating times so that they occurred within an eight- to eleven-hour window for four months, they lost eight pounds and kept it off. A control group that had no time restrictions on their eating lost no weight or *gained* weight. The researchers were confused—they hadn't asked any of the subjects to limit or change the foods they were eating in any way, but it was clear that eating within a shorter window of time improved health. What the authors had unintentionally created was something that mimicked an ancient technique we know as fasting.

One of the things we're learning about fasting is that it was actually a natural practice of our ancestors in times when food was scarce. It's also been used as a religious observance. The human body is not only made to endure fasting but thrives on it. Why? Because fasting lowers insulin (which stops fat storage), it increases metabolism (which makes you burn more calories), and it gives your body the time it needs *not eating* to do all sorts of repairing and rejuvenation to your cells that it normally can't do because of all the food you throw down your gullet. Fasting is actually the oldest and most effective lifestyle practice that helps you to lose excess weight and to maintain a healthy weight—and better health overall.

Understanding the Factory Inside You

You've heard about metabolism—you know, "your calorie-burning engine." Usually, you hear that metabolism is something you want to rev up to burn off more calories to lose weight faster. This really only touches the surface of what your metabolism does.

"Metabolism" is a blanket term used to represent *all* of the biochemical reactions that take place inside every one of the trillions and trillions of cells that constitute your body. These chemical reactions are occurring at every second to keep your body and brain alive and functioning properly. A highly functioning metabolism means a super-healthy and happy you.

That doesn't mean that you just want to have the fastest metabolism possible. Why? Mark Sisson, the founder of Primal Nutrition and Primal Kitchen and author of *The Primal Blueprint,* is a good friend and mentor whom I've known for more than a decade. When I recently talked to Sisson, he brought up the fact that hummingbirds have extremely fast metabolisms and live on average just three to five years, while animals like elephants have slow ones and can live for sixty to seventy years. "This tells you that a too-fast or a *hyper*-metabolism isn't necessarily better for your health or longevity. You don't want your metabolism to be stuck at one extreme or the other. You want an engine that is finely tuned, highly efficient, and operating at its peak performance level," says Sisson.

PATHWAYS OF EATING

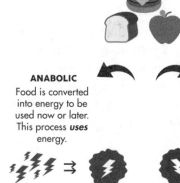

When we eat, food is diverted to one of two pathways:

ANABOLIC
Food is converted into energy to be used now or later. This process **uses** energy.

CATABOLIC
Stored fat is broken down so it can be used as fuel. This process **releases** energy.

Think of a large orchestra that masterfully plays Beethoven's Fifth Symphony (you know, "Da-Da-Da-DUMMM"). Your body's metabolism can be compared to an orchestra because it harmonizes many metabolic processes (instruments) that occur in your body. These processes boil down into two basic pathways: One takes the food you eat (the protein, carbs, and fats) and transforms it into energy that can be stored or excreted as waste (the anabolic pathway). The second is the process that breaks the molecules of stored energy back down for your body to use as fuel (the catabolic pathway).

The orchestra's job is to make the music beautiful. Therefore, the result the conductor seeks is a highly efficient, finely tuned orchestra (metabolism), not one with some musicians who play too fast while others are too slow. You don't want discord and chaos—or a strong desire for some earplugs. What we want is absolute synchronicity!

METABOLISM ORCHESTRA

When your metabolism is in perfect balance, it's like beautiful music. When it's sluggish or out of "tune" it produces a racket.

| BALANCED METABOLISM | UNBALANCED METABOLISM |

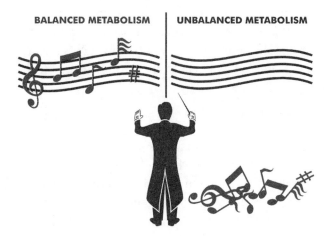

In our society, the reality of the situation is that most of us struggle with an ever-slower metabolism—one that could use some revving up. Just know that when I say, "Rev your metabolism," I'm talking about tuning your metabolism to its optimum speed. To do this requires you to eat the right foods at the right times, but also to understand your personal metabolism.

Charging Up Your Calorie-Burning Engine

You are one of a kind, and if you want to power up your metabolism so that it is a fat-burning machine, it is essential that you understand your personal metabolism and how it works. Researchers still don't have a definitive answer for why some people can eat with abandon and stay slim and fit while others (most of us) can't. What scientists do recognize is that we all have a distinct chemical design and each person's metabolism is dynamic. That's good news because it means that your metabolism can be changed by when and what you eat, how you move, and how you sleep.

If you have low energy and excess weight, it's safe to bet that you have a sluggish metabolism. If you are always anxious and restless, you could have an overactive thyroid, which accelerates your metabolism. Both could be influenced by the genes you inherit from your parents, their parents, and their parents' parents. One person from a certain genetic, cultural, or even ethnic background will metabolize food at a different rate from someone else. It's all good. The metabolic hand you've been dealt, as well as your current metabolism (the one you've influenced with poor eating habits, lack of sleep, too much stress, and not enough physical activity), is about to change. Cruise Control is going to show you how to make simple changes to your eating habits that are delicious, fully satisfying, *and* that will help to rev up your metabolism.

What Not to Eat

Okay. It's time for you to understand how *not* to eat.

All parts of your body (your brain, muscles, heart, and liver) need energy (from food) to function effectively. Feed your body the right foods and increase your energy and mood. You'll tune up your metabolism, burn fat, maintain a healthy weight, be healthier, happier, more serene, and you'll live longer. Feed your body the wrong foods, and your metabolism and energy will be stuck in the slow lane behind one of those Sunday drivers. The wrong foods will cause your arteries to harden and clog up (think French fries and chips), which increases your risk of high blood pressure and heart disease. The bad foods also make you unhealthy and overweight. And wait, there's more: eating the wrong foods gives you brain fog, throws off concentration, and makes you look older faster (that's why you wake up all bloated and puffy-looking after a night of KFC). Also, in addition to spiking insulin, eating high-sugar foods increases natural opioids and dopamine in your brain (these are the same chemicals found in highly addictive drugs). Eating foods that are high in sugar can cause you to excessively crave and binge on ever more high-sugar foods. Finally, your gut bacteria, the organs that make up your entire digestive system, are damaged by eating highly processed and high-sugar foods.

How the Wrong Foods Beat You Down

I'm going to say it again: Insulin is the hormone that tells your body to store fat. This hormone is signaled any time you eat, especially if you eat lots of carbs. If you eat a turkey sandwich, the bread causes sugar in your blood to increase, and this signals insulin, which quickly tells your body what to do with the food and where it should go—it can either be used immediately, put into your muscles and liver, or stored as fat all over your body. Interestingly, while protein does not spike blood sugar as carbs do, when you eat protein your pancreas still gets the signal to secrete insulin. What does this mean? It means that you want to eat moderate amounts of protein, not the levels that are prescribed in some keto diets. Cruise Control has got your back! As you'll see, we'll be keeping your carbs to 30 percent per day and your protein at 20 percent, and therefore keeping you in a safe fat-burning zone.

If you are eating too many sugars (remember all carbs are actually a version of sugar), it reprograms your body to store more and more fat. Did you hear me? Too much sugar (from carbs) causes too much insulin, and all of that makes your body change sugar into fat.

Weirdly, when your body thinks it is starving, it stores up excessive fat. When your fat stores build up too much, it prevents insulin from working properly in your liver. Your liver then tells your pancreas to release glucagon, a hormone that is supposed to counteract insulin. In a healthy person, this would signal your body to break down stored fats to use them for energy. However, if you are overweight or obese, or suffering from a related condition, the glucagon turns on gluconeogenesis, which actually makes more glucose (sugar). When this happens, the whole miserable cycle starts again: your insulin is triggered, and you store up more and more fat. Insulin spikes so much that your body starts

THE VICIOUS CYCLE

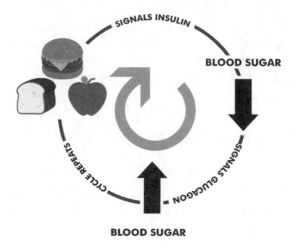

to store fat where it shouldn't, like your liver and muscles. And round and round it goes, and rounder and rounder you become.

Eating a diet that is too high in carbs and sugars will ruin your metabolic processes. When researchers followed more than 120,000 men and women for over twenty years, they found that those who consumed the most sugary beverages, starchy veggies (think potatoes and corn), refined grains (most bread and pasta), and processed foods had the biggest trouble with excess weight and obesity, compared to those who ate less of these foods. The study, published in the *New England Journal of Medicine,* also found that these fat-causing foods were less filling (so the people who ate them were hungrier and ate more) than high-fiber, healthy-fat, protein, low-carb diets. The bottom line: If you eat a high-carb, low-fat, processed diet you will probably gain weight, which will lead to an increased risk of all the chronic diseases I've already mentioned numerous times, and this will shorten your life. Plus, you'll never feel satisfied because your body will constantly tell you that it's starving and needs more food.

One last thing about processed foods, and why eating them is one of the worst things you can do to your body. Think about a bag of Doritos or a sandwich on white bread with turkey lunch meat and a slice of American cheese (don't forget the mayo). Thanks to the preservatives in these processed foods, eating them is—in metabolic terms—more "thermodynamically efficient." That sounds like a good thing, right? It's not!

Thermodynamically efficient means that your body doesn't need to use the energy it should to digest the food. The refining process that these processed foods go through strips out vitamins, fiber, nutrients, minerals, and natural antioxidants. What's left is not a lot of energy for your body to use or digest—just empty calories. You might as well eat sawdust.

If you want to unleash the full force of your metabolism, you're going to need to fuel your engine with foods that will bring your metabolism back to peak performance.

The Cruise Control eating plan is designed to clean out, build up, and rev up your engine by providing you with the best fuel for your body. I do this by incorporating Boost (time-restricted eating) and Burn (intermittent fasting) Zones that maximize how you burn the stored fat in your body while *minimizing* the amount of fat you store on your body in the first place. You'll learn all about Boost and Burn Zones and how they work in the next chapter. The result is a beautiful, sleek, and sexy running (and looking) machine.

LINDA **CARLSON**

AGE: 56 | WEIGHT LOST: 21 POUNDS

What everyone needs to know: You can lose two sizes on Cruise Control. That's what happened to me. I've lost so much weight that I keep having to "retire" items from my wardrobe. I have a little private celebration every time something that I couldn't even button a few weeks ago is now falling off of me because it's so loose.

THE SCIENCE OF
TIME-RESTRICTED EATING

If you're interested in the wealth of groundbreaking science behind the many health benefits of my Cruise Control program, check out Appendix A, page 283. Here's what we know about less frequent eating:

EATING LESS FREQUENTLY HELPS YOU KEEP OFF WEIGHT. A 2010 study in the *British Journal of Nutrition* found that participants who ate three meals and three snacks per day had no greater weight loss than those who ate just three meals per day, calories being equal. "Grazing" did nothing for weight loss.

EATING LESS FREQUENTLY BOOSTS YOUR STAY-YOUNG, LEAN-MUSCLE HORMONES. Scientists at the Intermountain Medical Center in Utah asked participants to fast for twenty-four hours and then compared their blood samples to those taken after a day of normal eating. They discovered that the male participants' levels of human growth hormone (HGH)—which protects lean muscle and regulates metabolism—were twenty times higher on the days when they fasted.

EATING LESS FREQUENTLY MAINTAINS MUSCLE FUNCTION. A 2012 research review in the *Journal of Sports Sciences* found that athletes who maintain their total energy and macronutrient intake, training load, body composition, and sleep length and quality are unlikely to suffer any substantial decrease in performance during fasting for Ramadan, the Muslim religious observance. And a 2011 study in the journal *Obesity Reviews* found that while intermittent fasting had the same effect on weight loss and fat loss as simply cutting calories, intermittent fasting seemed to be more effective for retaining lean muscle mass.

The Body-Fat Basement Freezer Model

In his book *The Complete Guide to Fasting,* Dr. Jason Fung compares glycogen, or sugar, to a refrigerator and your body fat to a basement freezer. Just like the refrigerator in your kitchen, your glycogen has a small freezer space where it can store a set amount of energy in the form of glucose. Your body fat is like a dedicated freezer in your basement that allows you to stock up on energy in much larger quantities, but it's also more of a hassle for you to carry the energy (food) from the basement up to your kitchen to thaw. It's such a pain to lug that food up those stairs that you won't bother with it if you have plenty of food in your fridge. In the same way, if you have glycogen (food in the fridge), you won't use the fat (food in the freezer).

BODY-FAT "BASEMENT FREEZER" MODEL

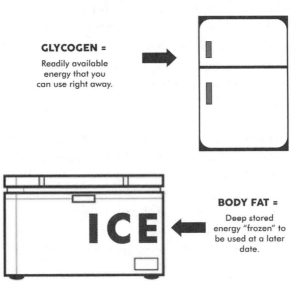

GLYCOGEN =
Readily available
energy that you
can use right away.

BODY FAT =
Deep stored
energy "frozen" to
be used at a later
date.

THE HISTORY OF FASTING

Of course, our ancestors didn't know they were fasting, they just ate according to the natural availability of food and light, and didn't eat in response to its scarcity. For more than 99 percent of our history on this planet, humans had to hunt and forage for their food. Availability and predictability of food weren't a given—let alone a drive-through Starbucks or a twenty-four-hour Dunkin' Donuts. It wasn't until ten thousand years ago that we began to settle into homesteads and farm—and bring food to us, instead of our going to the food. As we developed as agricultural societies, our periods of famine decreased, and over time we discovered ways of preserving, transporting, and providing foods until our 24/7 eating patterns of today developed. Where we once ate produce that came only at certain times of the year with certain seasons, today we can even have tropical fruit in winter.

We can trace the history of fasting back to ancient civilizations such as the Greeks, who practiced purposeful periods of time without food. At that time, fasts were believed to be strategies for cleansing, detoxifying, and purifying the body—and you can trace fasting as a spiritual and healing tradition that is still used in all major religions today. Three of the most influential men in the history of the world, Jesus Christ, Buddha, and the Prophet Muhammad, all shared a common belief in the healing power of fasting. In spiritual terms, it is often called "cleansing" or "purification," but practically, it amounts to the same thing. Here are a few examples of spiritual fasting from ancient traditions that are still used today:

- **Ramadan**: In Islam, during the month of Ramadan, Muslims observe a complete fast from dawn to dusk. This ritual is meant to focus one's attention on gratitude for the Creator.
- **Yom Kippur**: In the Jewish tradition, Yom Kippur is the Day of Atonement. Observers abstain from eating, drinking, bathing, washing, and sex. Yom Kippur is a twenty-five-hour fast, practiced as a time of "spiritual cleansing." The fast time is to be spent focusing on atonement and introspection.
- **Lent**: In the Christian and Catholic traditions, Lent is a forty-day period of total fasting (not intermittent or daytime), which makes it a little different from what we've been discussing. Today, most observers of Lent don't go all-in but rather abstain from certain foods—sweets or alcohol or meat or whatever it is one decides to give up during the forty-day period.
- **Hinduism**: Fasting is an integral part of the Hindu tradition, and it is often incorporated daily, weekly, and monthly. Each fast day focuses on a different deity. Usually, one picks a day of the week and doesn't eat until the afternoon. One can have water. In the afternoon one may eat a couple of pieces of fruit and some fruit juice. It's believed that if one sacrifices a day of eating, one's sins will be lessened.

- **Upavasa:** In some Buddhist traditions monks will fast for many days at a time as a way to purify the body and cleanse thoughts. During Upavasa (the period of fasting), only a small amount of water is allowed. At the end of the fast, the practitioner eats porridge.

The takeaway: Fasting is thousands of years old, and it is still practiced all over the world. You can practice this ancient technique with my modern spin to get all the benefits of intermittent fasting without the downsides.

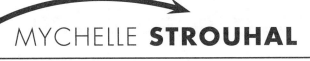

MYCHELLE **STROUHAL**

AGE: 49 | WEIGHT LOST: 20 POUNDS

What everyone needs to know: This is not a diet, it really is a lifestyle! Cruise Control is incredibly easy to follow, and you don't ever feel deprived. This plan also works for my family dynamic. I have a husband who travels 60 percent of each month, I work as a full-time realtor, and we have two active teens. Our schedules are moving targets, and I used to "survive" on feeding myself and my family fast food. Now my family helps to prepare for the week by having a weekend "grill" day where we grill up all our protein for the coming week. We also prep veggies, salads, and healthy snacks. I haven't had any fast food for over eight weeks, and I feel fabulous!

I no longer have carb comas or feel sluggish in the afternoon. I have unbelievable energy, increased motivation, stronger self-confidence, improved blood pressure, and reduced hot flashes. My doctor is thrilled with the progress I've made, and of course, I love that I can fit into all my favorite clothes that I haven't been able to wear for years. I've found a lifestyle that will keep me effortlessly Cruising on down the road to better health, and that's exactly what I'm going to do.

CHAPTER 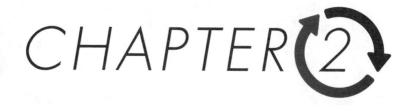 2

Turning On Cruise Control and Starting to Burn

A wise person considers that health
is the greatest of blessings.
— HIPPOCRATES

C ruise Control has allowed me—and countless others—to reap all the benefits of intermittent fasting with
none of the adverse side effects. Your body gets what it
needs to perform well without feeling hungry. Your
brain is energized, your mood is elevated, and you won't feel irritable. Cruise Control provides all the metabolic benefits of a fast.

What you'll see on Cruise Control is that you'll effortlessly melt
away flab, while forming a smooth and sculpted physique, even
with no exercise or calorie restriction. I saw my own six-pack surface while doing less training than I've ever done before. The bonus
is that using healthy fats as a morning strategy will help your body
shift from sugar burning to fat burning even if you've enjoyed

carbs the night before. Say goodbye to extreme carbohydrate restriction! Cruise Control increases ketones without complete carb cutting.

Ketogenic diets are nothing new, but Cruise Control is—I've discovered a *fast* hack that gives you the benefits of ketosis without any downside. Staying in ketosis for too long can cause constipation, low body temperature, bad breath, adrenal fatigue, and even an accumulation of biogenic histamines in the bloodstream. I also think that there's a misconception that keto lifestyles are for muscle-bound bodybuilding guys, not women. Not on Cruise Control! The combination of Burn and Boost Zones will cause your body to gently and safely dip in and out of ketosis, which powerfully battles metabolic conditions including diabetes, cancer, arthritis, Alzheimer's, and more.

Now that you know about the clockwork of eating, how insulin (not calories) makes you fat, and how metabolism *really* works, you are ready to take over the driver's seat on the journey to your best health with the Cruise Control Diet. It's time for you to learn about the components that make Cruise Control so effortlessly effective. Specifically, we're going to take a close look at dividing your day into two nutritional zones so that your body is always focused on boosting your metabolism and burning off unnecessary fat. These are your Burn and Boost Zones. In these next pages, I'm going to break it all down and give you your road map for effectively and efficiently carving up your day into twenty-four-hour chunks of metabolism-revved peak performance.

I have never before witnessed a lifestyle strategy that transforms health so dramatically. Of the thousands of clients who are already dedicated Cruisers, I'm regularly hearing stories of twenty-pound weight loss in just two weeks, of being taken off blood pressure medication, of eliminating diabetes symptoms, and more. These folks are excited about slimming down and firming up, and they are equally excited about having clear and radiant skin, shiny and luxuriant hair, of feeling like they have the clarity and focus they haven't felt for years. You're about to learn how weight loss and fat burning are just the tip of the iceberg when it comes to Cruise Control.

THE FOUR STEPS TO TURN ON CRUISE CONTROL

The Cruise Control program combines ancient dietary wisdom with modern nutritional science. What's unique about Cruise Control is the multifaceted approach used to achieve total body transformation. You are going to incorporate strategies that address the psychological, physiological, genetic, and sociological components for a truly remarkable metamorphosis. In short, Cruise Control is a comprehensive approach to boost your overall well-being with four powerful secrets:

Step 1: Nutrient Timing: The secret weapon of Cruise Control is the consumption of food nutrients in rhythm with your body's burning (fasting) and boosting (eating) cycles. I believe this is a missing link to building a healthy body and cleansing it of unwanted toxins and stubborn fat. By consuming solid foods within a finite window of time each day, your body is able to fully utilize the nutrients you eat and to cleanse, recharge, repair, and restore.

On Cruise Control, you'll eat Boost Zone foods during an eight-hour window each day. You already know that the average American eats for fifteen or more hours of the day. We're simply flipping the script. It's so incredibly simple and straightforward. Instead of grazing for the majority of the day, after your eight hours are completed, you'll enjoy healthy and satisfying Burn Zone beverages, snacks, and treats during the other sixteen hours of the day. These strategies will give your body the time it needs to clean, repair, and recharge itself.

It boils down to this: you'll eat during the eight-hour time of the day that works for you (see "Choose Your Window," below). It really doesn't matter other than choosing a time that works with your schedule.

CHOOSE YOUR WINDOW

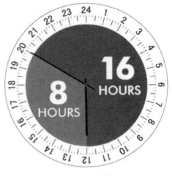

Your goal on Cruise Control is to follow the Boost Zone for an eight-hour window of time during the day and then to stick to the Burn Zone rules for the other sixteen hours of the day and night. What's important is choosing a time that works best for your lifestyle.

- **11:00 A.M. to 7:00 P.M.** If you want to eat dinner with your family later in the evening, you can schedule your Boost Zone to end at a time when you normally have an evening meal. Remember, you'll still enjoy your Cruise Control Coffee and other Burn Zone treats early in the morning, but you'll break your Burn in late morning.

- **7:00 A.M. to 3:00 P.M.** Alternately, if you're a morning person who loves breakfast but isn't big on dinner, you might choose to have your Boost Zone meals earlier. Here you break your Burn with your first Boost meal at seven in the morning. In this case, your last meal would end at three in the afternoon.

- **9:00 A.M. to 5:00 P.M.** If you have a little wiggle room for dinner but don't want to wait until later to break your fast, this time might be best for you.

- **Going for a Super Burn:** If you have a day when you find yourself not feeling hungry, feel free to Burn longer than sixteen hours. The longer you *Burn*, the more fat burning you'll see. I practice a twenty-four hour fast two to three times a week to detoxify my body and reset my gut. It's not as hard as it sounds because you still get to eat each day. I will often eat dinner at 6:00 P.M., and then eat dinner at 6:00 P.M. the following day. In between, I still enjoy Burn Zone treats. You can also do lunch to lunch, or any other time of the day that appeals. Simple, right? You eat one Boost Zone meal on day one, then you Burn until day two at the same time. You still eat in the Boost Zone daily, but just once on each day. You are in the driver's seat (more details on Super Burning on page 137).

- **Going to the Oscars?** Dinner won't be until 8:00 P.M. or later? Just shift your window to ensure a sixteen-hour Burn after the fancy festivities!

Step 2: Manipulate Your Nutrients: On Cruise Control you'll be manipulating your macronutrient intake at different times of the day to ignite your body's natural fat-burning ability and boost your metabolism. How? More on this in the next chapter, but here's the short version:

- You'll eat a wide variety of delicious foods abundant in healthy fats and oils.
- You'll enjoy moderate amounts of the highest-quality protein.
- You'll eat a reasonable amount of yummy, healthy, nutrient-dense, and carbohydrate-containing foods.

Burning at a Glance: During the sixteen-hour Burn Zone, you'll enjoy treats and beverages made of 100 percent healthy fats. Following this protocol will restrict the amount of glucose you consume, cutting off the glucose supply to your cells, lowering insulin levels, and ultimately forcing your body to burn fat for fuel.

BURN ZONE MACROS

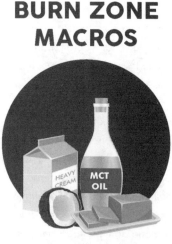

100% FAT

Boosting at a Glance: During the eight-hour Boost Zone, your diet will consist of 50 percent fat, 30 percent carbohydrates, and 20 percent protein. This breakdown of nutrients helps your body to rev up your metabolism and to pump up your health and vitality. Don't bother with your calculator. I've done all the math for you.

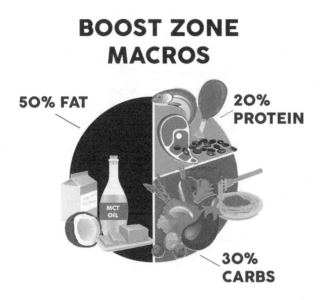

BOOST ZONE MACROS

50% FAT

20% PROTEIN

30% CARBS

Step 3: Friendly Fats: Medium-chain triglycerides (MCTs) are a form of saturated fatty acids that come with many health benefits including increased brain function and healthy weight management. Coconut oil is a top source of MCTs, comprised of nearly 65 percent of total fatty acids. This type of fat produces four times more brain-friendly energy in the form of ketones compared to regular coconut oil. MCTs are also called medium-chain fatty acids (MCFAs) and are largely missing from our industrialized diets. Why? Because the public has been misled to believe that all forms of saturated fats are potentially harmful. Quite the contrary, as compared to other types of oils and fats, MCTs seem to have positive effects on fat burning and weight reduction. As part of a healthy diet, MCTs and coconut oil can help increase satiety and even raise the metabolic rate at which the body functions. Since you will be fasting for sixteen hours a day, it's essential that you embrace these healthy fats as your friends.

Step 4: Caffeine: I have developed a delicious recipe for Cruise Control Coffee (or tea) that is filled with energizing antioxidants and caffeine, and all the best healthy fats you need to stay satisfied and revved up all day long (see page 37 in this chapter or a detailed recipe and options in chapter 6). Additionally, I recommend organic food sources of caffeine combined with powerful antioxidants such as green and black tea (unsweetened) to give you that extra boost of energy as you begin to transition from your current eating habits. Caffeine can help with a temporary lack of energy. In addition, having your coffee in the morning can be an especially helpful fuel for your brain. Research shows that a breakfast cup of coffee can increase ketones, the brain-friendly energy produced when your insulin levels are low enough. Scientific studies also show that caffeine defends against cognitive decline and reduces the risk of Alzheimer's disease, and it increases insulin sensitivity in healthy humans, which is extremely important to sustained weight loss. Why does it boost your mood? Coffee may alter serotonin and dopamine activity for a short-term emotional boost, while the antioxidants and anti-inflammatory compounds in coffee have been linked to long-term effects on mood.

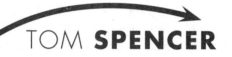

TOM **SPENCER**

AGE: 44 | WEIGHT LOST: 41 POUNDS

What everyone needs to know: I can bend over and tie my own shoes! That might sound like no great feat, but I couldn't do this a few weeks ago. I can also now cut my lawn without needing to take breaks at the end of each row, and have lost three sizes. I had a few times where the scale froze up on me, but the support from other Cruisers helped me to not give in to the old habits of popping junk in my cake-hole. The on-line support has been incredible.

UPGRADE YOUR CRUISE CONTROL WITH MY COFFEE, BARS, AND SHAKE!

Over the past two years that I've been writing and developing this book, I've been in search of some instant and easy way to carry coffees and on-the-go meals that come with all the power of healthy fats and other Cruise Control ingredients. I've found some good instant coffees, but not any that have the healthy fats, the minerals, and that are made with organic coffee beans in the exact concentrations that fit the specifications of Cruise Control. So, I developed my own! I worked with one of the world's leading nutrition manufacturers to develop exactly the products I'd envisioned. You can find information about my Cruise Control products, including my coffee, fat bars, and my healthy fat shake, in the Resources section, page 302.

First I knew we needed healthy fats to keep my clients in the Burn Zone, so that meant organic grass-fed butter and healthy MCTs, but how do you get powdered butter and oil? We did it. Our powdered butter is made from pasture-raised, grass-fed, antibiotic- and hormone-free cows. This type of butter contains butyrate, a fatty acid that helps your gut by promoting digestion. Next, we took MCTs made from pure coconut oil and designed a powder version. These two healthy fats are used in my coffee, bars, and shakes to keep you in a fat-burning fasted state but without any of the downsides of fasting (hunger, irritability, or fatigue). MCTs and coconut oil are also known to boost your brain health and help you maintain a healthy weight.

By including organic Himalayan pink salt and the best organic, fair-trade, instant coffee, you get the minerals and healthy caffeine you need to boost your energy and mental focus. Himalayan pink salt helps your body to be in electrolyte balance to aid calorie burning, promote healthy circulation, and better absorb nutrients. This all adds up to a balanced metabolism, a healthy gut, and all the benefits of fasting without spiking your blood sugar or signaling your insulin. That means that you keep burning stored fat that is currently on your body. Here are the results of my work and research:

- Cruise Control Instant Organic Coffee: This delicious instant fair-trade coffee tastes like it was made from freshly ground beans. You'll get a nice

150 mg of caffeine per serving (comparable to a 12-ounce cup of coffee) to provide a boost in the morning or pick-me-up to get you through the day without leaving you overly jittery. The grass-fed butter and MCTs from coconut oil will keep you energized and feeling full while burning fat, and the Himalayan salt will help your metabolism stay balanced, so you keep humming along.

- Cruise Control Creamer: If you prefer to still order your venti dark roast at you-know-where, no worries. I was also able to develop and design my own Cruise Control–approved healthy-fat creamer that you can add to your coffee or favorite tea. This blend is also made from coconut oil, grass-fed butter, and MCTs that will help you feel energized and satisfied, and you'll stay in a fat-burning state. You'll enhance your brain's favorite form of energy, ketones, which have been shown to boost cognitive clarity and focus. There's also Himalayan pink salt with more than eighty minerals that promote healthy circulation and a balanced metabolism to keep you feeling your best.

- Cruise Control Fat Bars: When you are on the go and dashing from place to place it can be hard to be prepared with a Boost Zone Meal at all times. I've designed a Cruise Control–approved meal replacement bar for just this situation. I always throw one in my bag. My bars provide fat-burning MCT oils, healthy protein, but keep carbs low. Plus, they are full of rich real chocolate and 10 grams of protein for just 270 calories.

- Cruise Control Fat Shake: My Cruise Control Coffee can be added to this delicious chocolate shake for an extra jolt of healthy energy, or you can enjoy its chocolatey goodness all on its own. It's also kid-friendly (my son Parker loves this shake). Here you get all the healthy MCT fats and Himalayan salt that are in my coffee and bars, and there are also collagen peptides for healthy bones and 10 grams of healthy protein from free-range eggs. Plus, you'll get other healthy fats from avocados, flaxseeds, and chia seeds (these are also fiber-rich and full of omega-3 fatty acids). At 220 calories and zero grams of sugar, this makes a perfect meal replacement while keeping you in the fat-burning zone.

You can find information for all products in the Resources section, page 302.

THE BURN ZONE: FASTING WITH FAT

Your Sixteen-Hour Window

In the Burn Zone (the "fasting with fat" phase), you will enjoy coffee, tea, and other approved items—and you will sleep. Together this will account for sixteen hours of your day, and since you'll be sleeping (hopefully for eight of those hours) you'll only have four hours in the morning and four hours in the evening when you might really want or need my Burn Zone treats. I call these four-hour blocks your "Bumper Zones" because this can initially be the time in which you *feel* most hungry. See more about Bumper Zones below.

Once you get past the first week of Cruise Control, chances are you won't even feel hungry during the Burn Zone bumper times, and you might even decide to forgo Burn Zone foods entirely—that's what most of my clients experience. You'll save money and time because you'll be buying and preparing less food while devoting your energy and brain power to other areas of your life. There's incredible freedom that comes from putting your life on Cruise Control. Health-wise, you'll feel less bloated, more clearheaded, and lighter in mind and body.

BUMPER ZONES

These zones are a subset of Burn Zones. Bumper Zones are the time period before your first meal in the Boost Zone and the one after your final Boost meal of the day before you go to bed. Remember, eight hours of the sixteen-hour Burn Zone will be spent in restful slumber. The first Bumper Zone occurs during the first four hours after you awaken, and the last four occur after your final meal before bed. Most of us are conditioned to get hungry around mid-morning, and so you can feel pretty ravenous around this time. This is where Cruise Control Coffee, Tea, or any of the other Burn Zone–approved treats will save the day. The second Bumper Zone occurs after your dinner. Again, this is another common time that many of us are conditioned to experience hunger, but no worries. Make a decaf Cruise Control Coffee or Tea, or any other Burn Zone food, and you'll be good to go. Remember, you won't be triggering blood sugar or insulin, so your body will still "think" you are fasting, but you'll feel great.

BURN ZONE BENEFITS

Depriving your body of food for a certain period of time provides enormous physical and mental benefits. It makes sense from an evolutionary standpoint. For most of history, humans weren't eating three square meals a day, plus snacks. Instead, humans evolved in situations where there wasn't much food, and they learned to thrive when fasting. Nowadays, we don't have to hunt for food, we spend most of our days in front of computers, and we eat whenever we want, but that isn't how your body is designed to function. It's why we are a nation of fat. It doesn't have to be this way.

By following the Burn Zone, you'll:

- Lose weight
- Never feel hungry
- Increase energy
- Accelerate cellular repair and recycling (when your body consumes defective tissue to produce new parts)
- Reduce insulin resistance and type 2 diabetes
- Lower bad cholesterol
- Live longer
- Protect against Alzheimer's and Parkinson's
- Improve memory and brain function
- Make cells more resilient

NUTRIENTS IN THE BURN ZONE

Your primary objective in the sixteen-hour Burn Zone is to keep insulin levels low to avoid fat storage and weight gain. The best way to do this is to avoid carbs and protein (they both raise insulin) and to focus on consuming healthy fats. The good news is that I have created some delicious Burn Zone recipes that you can enjoy as much as you want. These recipes contain healthy fats, herbs, and spices that keep you in the fat-burning mode, while simultaneously boosting your energy and keeping you satisfied. You will *not* feel hungry during the Burn Zone. Prepare to be amazed.

CHEAT YOUR FAST WITH FAT

Cruise Control is *not* regular intermittent fasting; it's not a diet, either. You are not going to feel overly hungry, you'll burn fat, and you'll build sleek, sexy muscle. Cruise Control is a method that helps your body quickly change from burning sugars to burning fat. How? By tricking your body into a near-ketogenic state with the Burn Zone.

Traditional keto diets work by keeping carbohydrates under 20 grams a day (the lower, the better). Getting your body to switch to fat burning takes about a week of committed eating that consists of zero to less than 20 grams of carbs daily, moderate protein, and lots of fat. According to Leanne Vogel, author of *The Keto Diet,* the most accurate method for testing for ketosis is to get a blood test. You are in ketosis if your results are between 0.5 and 3.0 mmol/L for ketone bodies. This is a good indicator that your body is well on its journey to becoming a fat-burning machine. You can also test for ketosis with a breath test (if you are willing to dish out between $150 and $200 for a meter). Finally, there are urine strips available, but these are the least accurate. The good news is that there are alternatives to testing. Vogel suggests answering the following questions to do a self-check to see if you are acting ketosis-like.

1. You can skip meals without getting hangry.

2. Going three to five hours without a snack is easy.

3. You don't have carb cravings or feel hungry two to three hours after your last meal.

4. You naturally prefer high-fat foods or high-carb ones.

5. You have plenty of energy for exercise.

6. You no longer have an afternoon slump.

7. Your brain is clear and focused.

If you agree with three or more of these statements, there's a good chance that you are in ketosis.

Unfortunately, keto diets require a stringent and limiting method of eating that most people have a hard time following for a long period of time. The benefits are many: weight loss, fat burning, low appetite, and high energy—but the side effects can also be miserable, ranging from bad breath, nausea, and headaches to dizziness, brain fog, and fatigue. But nothing else burns off stubborn belly fat like a keto diet—until now.

The research is showing that if you can hit the lower ranges of ketosis, around 0.48 to 0.5, then it will make a huge difference in the amount of fat you burn. That's what you'll regularly do on Cruise Control. Your body will automatically dip into this range every twenty-four hours. What a difference that makes! You'll automatically reset your hunger hormone (ghrelin) and your satisfaction hormone, cholecystokinin (CCK).

How do you exceed that magic number, 0.48, to reset your hunger hormones and burn fat (which means you won't feel hungry, but you'll be shedding weight like crazy)? More important, how is it possible that Cruise Control allows carbohydrates every day and still gets this result?

By cheating your fast with fats! When you consume the right amount of coconut or MCT oil, within minutes your body processes these fats and your ketone levels can go into that magic Burn Zone. That means you'll have higher ketone levels than someone who eats carbs, but less than someone on a traditional ketogenic diet. Which means you won't have food cravings, and you'll feel full and satisfied because your hunger hormones will be turned down low. Amazing! Best of all, consuming only healthy fats without any protein or carbs means that your body essentially stays in a fasted state. Fat won't raise your insulin or cause your liver to deal with the demands of digestion. You'll get all of the benefits automatically without hitting any of the potholes.

CRUISE CONTROL VOCABULARY

The language you choose to use in your daily life can make a big difference in how you feel, what you think, and the actions you take. I'm a big believer in choosing the most positive and empowering words because I've seen first-hand how negative self-talk and words can tear someone down, and how using positive language can shift a person's intention from helpless to confident. With this in mind, I've reformulated the language around intermittent fasting to be more positive and empowering and also to be more accurate and factual.

- **Cruise Control:** My new and improved version of intermittent fasting or time-restricted eating (TRE).
- **Boost Zone:** This is the time of the day that you'll be refilling your energy stores with Boost Zone foods and meals that will boost your metabolism, reduce inflammation, keep you energized, and help you to feel your best.
- **Burn Zone:** This is the period of time that taps into your body's hidden potential, formerly known as fasting. During this sixteen-hour period, you are going to turn on your body's fat-burning machine.
- **Burn Zone Treats or Bumper Zone Foods:** Yummy, healthy, fat-rich treats and drinks that you can eat any time of day—when burning or boosting!

CRUISE CONTROL COFFEE

Cruise Control Coffee is much more than a venti latte. It's a high-performance beverage that has a massive impact on your energy and cognitive function. I've seen Cruise Control Coffee help countless people, from busy parents to professional athletes to celebrities, rev up energy and improve health. Here's the breakdown:

WHAT IS CRUISE CONTROL COFFEE?

1. It all starts with the beans. Brew 1 cup (8 to 12 ounces) of ground coffee using filtered water. You can also brew a cup of your favorite tea as a substitute for the coffee.

2. Add 1 teaspoon to 2 tablespoons of MCT or coconut oil. Start with 1 teaspoon per cup and work your way up to 1 to 2 tablespoons over several days.

3. Add 1 to 2 tablespoons of grass-fed, unsalted butter or 1 to 2 teaspoons of grass-fed ghee (for those who can't tolerate dairy). You read that right. It says butter. Don't worry. This mixture also makes the creamiest, most delicious cup of coffee you've ever had. Oh, and make sure your butter is unsalted.

4. Add a pinch of Himalayan pink salt to alkalize and flood the body with electrolytes.

5. Mix it all up with a spoon or blender for 20 to 30 seconds until it looks like a foamy latte.

Note: If your mixture is really hot, be careful opening up the blender before you pour.

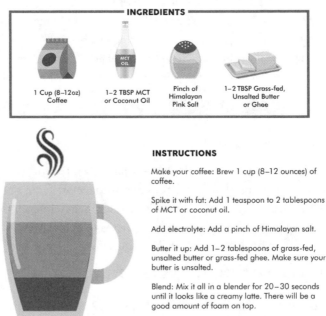

CRUISE CONTROL COFFEE

INGREDIENTS

| 1 Cup (8–12oz) Coffee | 1–2 TBSP MCT or Coconut Oil | Pinch of Himalayan Pink Salt | 1–2 TBSP Grass-fed, Unsalted Butter or Ghee |

INSTRUCTIONS

Make your coffee: Brew 1 cup (8–12 ounces) of coffee.

Spike it with fat: Add 1 teaspoon to 2 tablespoons of MCT or coconut oil.

Add electrolyte: Add a pinch of Himalayan salt.

Butter it up: Add 1–2 tablespoons of grass-fed, unsalted butter or grass-fed ghee. Make sure your butter is unsalted.

Blend: Mix it all in a blender for 20–30 seconds until it looks like a creamy latte. There will be a good amount of foam on top.

Starting your day with cereal, granola, oatmeal, toast, fruit, or another carb-heavy breakfast staple spikes your blood sugar. You'll get a quick burst of energy, but by mid-morning your blood sugar will crash, and you'll be hungry, tired, and unfocused. There's a better way to go: Cruise Control Coffee *is* breakfast—sans the insulin spike that causes fat storage or the crash that comes from eating foods such as fruits, smoothies, cereals, or other bread products. When your brain is running on fat instead of sugar, you have more focus and won't experience the drops in energy that come with a high-carb diet. Your metabolism will switch into fat-burning mode, which frees you from sudden energy crashes and brain fog.

Start your day with Cruise Control Coffee, for the following benefits:

- **Satisfaction and Serenity:** MCT or coconut oil balances ghrelin, the hormone that makes you want to eat, and CCK, the hormone that keeps you feeling full. Balancing and harmonizing these hormones means that you'll be steadily energized and focused, but not hungry or irritable. There are also some studies that show that a couple of cups of coffee a day can improve your mood and sense of alertness.

- **Strong, Stable Energy:** The saturated fat in grass-fed butter and ghee slows, but doesn't negate, the absorption of caffeine. Your body will process the energy over several hours, keeping you highly productive. You won't have the spikes, crashes, or jitters you can get from coffee alone or with sugar. MCT oil is a purified form of medium-chain triglyceride derived from 100 percent pure coconut oil. It's then triple-distilled through earthen clay, so there are no solvent residues.

- **A Sharp Mind:** Both MCT and coconut oil rapidly convert to ketone bodies. These molecules are your brain's favorite because the energy they produce is more powerful than what comes from sugars. Coffee is packed with essential nutrients like B vitamins, potassium, and manganese. Additionally, coffee is rich in antioxidants that protect your brain and body from the effects of memory loss and aging. Bioflavonoids in coffee can intensify neuronal firing in your brain and help brain cells communicate faster. That means that your thoughts come more quickly, and you'll have a sharper memory. Thanks to the one-two punch of ketones and caffeine, you'll literally feel your brain turning on.

- **Metabolic Boost:** Coffee increases your metabolism by up to 20 percent. Plain intermittent fasting doesn't. This combination is superior. Caffeine boosts physical endurance, which makes workouts feel effortless. The caffeine in coffee can also raise your metabolism to help you burn fat.
- **Better Nutrient Potency:** Your body craves good fats for hormone balance and brain health. But good-quality, grass-fed butter or ghee also contains omega-3 fatty acids, beta-carotene, fat-soluble vitamins A, D, E, and K, CLA (conjugated linoleic acid, a fatty acid with powerful fat-loss benefits), and antioxidants.
- **Pain and Inflammation Reduction:** Grass-fed butter is high in a short-chain fatty acid called butyrate that has been shown to both prevent and decrease inflammation.
- **More Intense Workouts:** Cruise Control Coffee makes an excellent fuel for fitness. Fueling with sugar and other simple carbs might give you a short-term spike, but it will leave you stranded in a slump during your workout.

NOT A COFFEE PERSON? NO WORRIES.

You can experience equal benefits by turning Cruise Control Coffee into Cruise Control Tea. Black and green teas still have caffeine and also have a compound that reduces stress. Research has shown that drinking tea revs up your metabolism and keeps you energized without the jitters that coffee can cause.

In fact, you can enjoy a creamy version of herbal teas, bone broth, and more by using the same healthy oils used in Cruise Control Coffee.

TUMMY TROUBLE

If you follow Cruise Control closely, the most common side effect will be feeling fantastic, but if you run into trouble, it's probably due to a couple of issues. If you are shifting from a low-fat, high-carb, restricted-calorie, or vegan diet (all insulin spiking), you might feel hungry when you first start your Burn Zone. This may tempt you to overindulge in the Burn Zone beverages and treats, and that can cause tummy trouble. Your body needs anywhere from a week to a month to fully switch to a fat-burning system. Eat too much fat too soon, and your belly may balk, and you may be running to the restroom more than you bargained for. MCT oil has the most powerful effects when it comes to a rumbling tummy—take it slow. Begin by adding as little as a teaspoon of MCT oil and increase from there. You can also provide your belly with extra protection by including a digestive enzyme before or during (not after) your drinks or meals. Look for a supplement that contains fat-digesting lipase and betaine HCl (betaine hydrochloride) because it will help better your stomach acid levels. It might take a few weeks to adjust, but it's worth it! Pretty soon you'll be feeling fantastic without any gut glitches.

Another possible issue could be that your stomach has weak levels of stomach acid, which can cause acid reflux. The correct level of stomach acid signals the valve that separates the esophagus from the stomach to stay closed. If you don't have enough to cause this switch to flip, your valve might not close—and then you may get—"urp," excuse me—indigestion troubles or acid reflux. Another problem that exacerbates acid reflux symptoms are the very medicines prescribed for the condition. These are called proton-pump inhibitors. The problem is that, while they work to temporarily stop heartburn, these medicines cause stomach acid to remain at dangerously low levels. That can mean that your stomach won't be able to kill off bad bacteria and toxins, and can ultimately result in serious bacterial infections. Using a digestive enzyme that contains betaine HCl won't do this because it increases stomach acid (which triggers your valve to close) and stops acid reflux. If you try this and you still have some gurgling, try mixing a teaspoon of baking soda in a small glass of water. This will neutralize existing excess acid without affecting overall levels as long as you don't make it a regular habit.

CHAPTER 3

Get a Boost: Eating Matters, Too

Eat to live, don't live to eat.
—BENJAMIN FRANKLIN

We've just discussed the power of adhering to a time-restricted eating pattern and allowing your body the time it needs to take a break from a focus on digestion during your sixteen-hour Burn Zone. But of course, you gotta eat, too! That's where the Boost Zone comes in.

THE EIGHT-HOUR BOOST ZONE

During a daily eight-hour window of your choice, you'll eat your main meals, made of Boost Zone–approved food. This eight-hour Boost Zone (the metabolism-boosting phase) may feel like a *long* time to eat two meals and snacks, and if you decide that five or six hours is more to your liking, more power to you! However, the research that looks at time-restricted eating shows that eight hours will provide you with all the effortless weight loss, fat burning, and metabolism-revving benefits you desire. The Boost Zone time turns food into high-octane fuel that will work like the best medicine available to your body. You'll enjoy a wide and delicious range of healthy fats, protein, and carbohydrates. You can see the breakdown of your macros in the Boost Zone food pyramid below. Remember, your macros will be 50 percent fat, 30 percent carbohydrates, and 20 percent protein. You can adjust your Boost and Burn Zones to times that work for you, based on your lifestyle (see "Choose Your Window," page 27). While 10:00 A.M. to 6:00 P.M. might be optimal for me, noon to eight at night might be better for you. The most important element is that you restrict your main meals to an eight-hour period of time.

BOOST ZONE FOOD PYRAMID

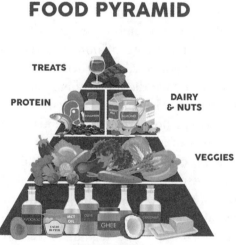

TREATS

PROTEIN

DAIRY & NUTS

VEGGIES

HEALTHY FATS

BOOST ZONE BENEFITS

Thanks to the high-carb, low-fat diet that most people follow, it's estimated that around 99 percent of Americans are sugar burners instead of fat burners. Remember, even a diet that includes moderate amounts of carbs will spike your insulin and encourage your body to store fat. You'll change that with Cruise Control. You're about to become the driver to your best health. Consider the following benefits:

- No food cravings or hunger
- Balanced hormones
- Effortless weight loss
- Enhanced mental clarity, focus, and concentration
- Amplified feelings of happiness and well-being
- Steady and strong energy
- Balanced blood sugar
- Improved insulin sensitivity
- Lowering of (bad) cholesterol and triglycerides
- Revved metabolism
- Healthy digestion
- Fortified immunity
- Reduced inflammation

That last one—reduced inflammation—is really critical. When I recently spoke with the world-famous Dr. Andrew Weil, he emphasized the importance of eating an anti-inflammatory diet.

"Inflammation is so powerfully destructive to the brain and body. It's at the root of cardiovascular disease, coronary artery disease, neurodegenerative diseases like Alzheimer's and Parkinson's, and cancer," he said. To reduce inflammation, Weil recommends a diet that's rich in vegetables, low amounts of animal protein, whole grains, less fruit, and olive oil as the main cooking oil. He added: "I also recommend anti-inflammatory spices such as ginger and turmeric, red wine and chocolate in moderation, and green tea." This eating plan will provide you with more physical and mental energy than ever before. Your mind will regain clarity and focus. Plus, you're going to feel more joyful, enthusiastic, confident, serene, and empowered. Oh, and you'll reap the little ole bonus of *living longer*.

All of that means that you'll be getting amazing, lasting benefits for your health—and your waistline. *Hel-low-oh!* or *"¡Pon atención!"* as my grandma would say.

So, let's get into unpacking the nutrition logic of Cruise Control. I'm going to explain some specifics about the nutrients you'll be consuming, which will be simple and delicious (of course), and how breakfast is *not* necessarily the most important meal of the day. We'll close this topic by zeroing in on the foods that serve as the best fuel for your body. By the time you're done with this chapter, you'll be ready to start the Four-Week Plan that follows.

WHAT DOES HEALTHY EATING ON CRUISE CONTROL MEAN?

Relying on macronutrient-based guidelines or calorie counting makes eating like driving a big ole stick shift bus on a bumpy dirt road. It's far more complicated, cumbersome, uncomfortable, and ineffective than necessary. Cruise Control avoids all these pitfalls. And it's simple. You have only two speeds—Boost and Burn—and they are both automatic. That's because I've done the work for you. All you have to do is focus on eating certain delicious meals in one zone, and other decadent treats in the other. Easy.

That said, I still believe it is vitally important for you to know the rationale behind the design that makes Cruise Control so powerfully effective. It's the scientifically proven strategies that will keep your motor running at top speed.

I've already soapboxed your ears about consistently high insulin levels being the source of our fat and chronic disease woes that add up to metabolic syndrome. And *not eating* is the best way to lower insulin, which is why fasting is showing a powerful resurgence. Of course, you can't just stop eating forever, and besides, who would want to do such a thing? Food is delicious. Thankfully, there's no need. There are far more delicious and enjoyable ways to keep your insulin levels consistently low. And thanks to the Cruise Control loophole of fasting with healthy fat, you'll never feel starved or depleted. Nope, you'll run like a race car.

I am not about suffering. I am about simple, effective results. And like my friend and self-proclaimed health detective Dr. Daryl Gioffre says, "The focus needs to be on what a food does inside your body once it has been metabolized." That's what I've done with Cruise Control.

THE CRUISE CONTROL RULES OF EATING

- **Eat Whole, Unprocessed Foods:** Just eat real food. Hey, this doesn't mean that every item you put in your mouth needs to be handpicked from your backyard organic garden. I'm a realist, and while I do believe that we humans are designed to eat whole, unprocessed, unpreserved, natural foods, I also know that it's nearly impossible to avoid all foods that come in packages, bottles, jars, bags, or boxes. Fortunately, today you can find frozen and boxed products that are natural and unrefined. The ingredient lists and nutrient labels of these items still make the cut as being "real food." The items that hurt our modern-day diets are those that are made with highly processed, refined sugars and flours, and the ones that come packed with preservatives, artificial colors, chemicals, processed fats, and lots and lots of complicated additives including things like butylated hydroxyanisole, sulfates, and benzoates. These are the "foods" that cause disease. The human brain and body are constructed to digest and absorb natural foods such as cooked proteins, whole greens, and unrefined vegetable fats. The human brain and body are not able to adequately digest and absorb Frankenstein foods (the ones it takes a laboratory to create). If you're grabbing food that is packaged, take a minute to read the ingredients. Are they recognizable as something that was alive, was picked off a plant or tree, or came out of the ground? That's what you want from your food. (As much as I've dreamed of it, I've never actually seen a tree that grows glazed doughnuts.)
- **Avoid Sugars and Refined Grains:** Yes, I'm repeating myself, but it's worth restating. While many packaged foods pass the Cruise Control quota, sugars and refined grains crash and burn every time. "I think the most important rule I would give people to start with is to avoid drinking sweet liquids," says Dr. Weil. "If we could just get people to stop drinking sweetened beverages and not as much soda, energy drinks, fruit juices, and sugary coffees and teas, we'd be a big step ahead on the obesity epidemic."

- **Eat More Natural Fats:** For decades, fat was the f-word in the nutrition world. Not anymore. Today, we know that we get many positive benefits from natural dietary fats for energy, nutrient absorption, cell repair, brain function, nerve processing, muscle movement, and reduction of inflammation and pain, and that's just a sampling. I'll be going into dietary fats in great detail in the next section of this chapter, so for now suffice it to say that your best friends in the fat world are extra-virgin, unrefined, organic, and cold-pressed olive oil, avocado oil, and coconut oil; raw nuts; avocados; fatty fish; grass-fed red meats; and grass-fed butter.
- **Eliminate Artificial Fats:** There are still bad fats, and you should avoid them at all times. At the top of this list are canola, safflower, and palm oil, and anything that says it is "partially hydrogenated," which means that a liquid oil has been chemically processed to turn it into solid fat. This includes refined vegetable oils, shortening, deep-fried foods, margarine, and baked goods such as cookies and cakes. These are trans fats and eating them is like eating plastic. Your body and your brain are not constructed to digest and absorb these foods. These fats raise "bad" cholesterol and lower your "good" cholesterol, increasing the risk of heart disease and stroke. This includes oils that we only recently considered to be "heart healthy," such as corn, soy, sunflower, and canola oils. Studies suggest that these oils are highly concentrated in inflammation-causing omega-6 fats. A small amount of omega-6 fats are part of a healthy diet, but today we eat around ten to twenty times more than we need. At the same time, we aren't getting omega-3 fats (found in fatty cold-water fish, nuts, and seeds). "The result is systemic inflammation which increases your risk of heart disease, type 2 diabetes, inflammatory bowel disease, and other chronic illnesses," says Weil.

DEBUNKING BREAKFAST

We've all heard the saying, "Breakfast is the most important meal of the day," but do you know the origin of it? Breakfast, lunch, dinner, and snacks are modern inventions, not genetically hardwired instincts such as hunger and survival.

What constitutes a breakfast and when did breakfast get its own designated foods?

Think about the word "breakfast." It's easy to see that it is a word that naturally morphed from the phrase "break the fast," to describe the first eating you do each day to break your nightly fast. Interestingly, the origin of the word comes from the Old English word for dinner, *disnar,* which means "to break a fast." However, in 1917 an article in *Good Health Magazine* took it a step further by stating, "In many ways, the breakfast is the most important meal of the day, because it is the meal that gets the day started." The editor of the magazine? None other than Dr. John Harvey Kellogg, the coinventor of many cold breakfast cereals (made of, by the way, highly refined grains). No surprise: In the 1980s and 1990s, cold cereal sales in the United States peaked (thanks, Dr. Kellogg).

I'm a big believer in science, but that doesn't mean that you can declare one study's findings from one point in time as a fact. When does something become a truth on which you can rely? It's debatable, but you can count on research findings a lot more when several studies have been published that look at increasing populations of people over an extended period of time. The majority of Americans today are more of a globe shape than an hourglass. Breakfast is part of this debacle because institutional interlopers that were and are highly motivated by money and politics such as the government and the food industry have had their way with us.

If you look at the fine print in hundreds, if not thousands, of studies that tout that breakfast is essential for health, nutrition, and weight loss, you'll see that they've been funded at least in part by companies such as Kellogg, Sara Lee, Oroweat, and others. You don't hear about these study sponsors in the media. The headlines tend to focus on the much sexier tidbits that refer to the findings that state that "those who regularly skip breakfast are 450 percent more likely to be obese," or the caution, "If you go for a period without eating, you'll lose muscle, not fat." The bummer is that it's simply not true. Thankfully, there are also plenty of studies (not funded by or promoting the food industry) that debunk these pro-breakfast "facts."

Consider a German study where investigators followed the eating habits of nearly three hundred obese participants and one hundred normal-weight participants. At the end of two weeks, the researchers found that both healthy weight and obese participants who ate the smallest morning meals (or no breakfast at all) consumed lower overall daily calories, while the more calories an individual ate for breakfast, the more total calories they ate during their entire day. These findings, which appeared in *Nutrition Journal* in 2011, suggest that a small meal or no breakfast at all might be the best way to reduce food intake. In fact, more and more research is proving that avoiding calories in the morning is the way to stay not only slim but also strong in both body and mind. In fact, this strategy can completely erase the damage of an otherwise "bad" diet.

BOOSTING YOUR NUTRITION

It's time to discuss how you'll fuel up, qualitatively, on Cruise Control to burn fat and harness the full potential of your metabolism. You are going to take control of those pesky insulin levels so you can synchronize all of your metabolic processes, which speed up your body's natural ability to burn fat, create energy, and fight disease. You're about to be introduced to the foods that will lower your blood sugar, increase your human growth hormone, and ramp up your metabolic rate by 14 percent. All of that means that you'll be effortlessly burning fat that is stored around your body. Let's take a look at each macronutrient.

Proteins

Look at your hand for a moment. You are looking at protein. Yep. Put protein under a microscope, and you'll see that it's made of various chains and configurations of amino acids that make up our human bodies. Proteins exist in every cell of your body, and they create the building blocks of you. Of course, there are other chemicals involved in what makes up you, but protein is the star when it comes to creating all the structures required in a working body; they build, maintain, and repair your bones, muscles, skin, cartilage, and more.

The building blocks of proteins? Those would be amino acids, which are the smaller units that link together to make unique shapes and functions of proteins. Amino acids are part of every metabolic process in your body, from transporting and storing nutrients, to protecting your immune system, to keeping your hair from falling out or your skin from wrinkling.

Where do the amino acids that make protein come from? Some are produced by your body from other sources, but mostly you get amino acids from the foods you eat. The process of digestion breaks down that protein-rich steak into the various amino acids that make it up. Then those acids go through a process that . . . would put you to sleep if I gave you all the chemistry mumbo-jumbo. Just know that amino acids reconstruct inside your body to create specific configurations to make shapes that make the proteins that make *you*. It's sort of like Legos. Let's say you had a Lego model of a drumstick, but you also have a Lego model of a person, and this Lego person's knee has been damaged. You'd first need to deconstruct the "drumstick," and then to reconfigure it to repair the Lego person's knee. That's an extremely simplified example of what goes on in your body, but it gives you an idea of how your body takes food apart so it can put it back together to repair, maintain, and make your body. Here are a few more things that proteins make possible in the human body:

- **Contentment:** Proteins are involved in the signaling in your brain that is triggered when you are full from a meal. These proteins interact with hormones in a multitiered way to let your brain and body know that it is satisfied, is in control, and no longer needs to eat.
- **Focus:** A lack of protein will signal a hormone that stimulates cravings. Cravings scatter your thinking so that you can't stay focused on your goals. If you eat lots of bread, crackers, and muffins, you may notice that you don't feel full and are soon thinking of how nice it would be to eat some more food. This is dangerous because it can cause you to overeat during your overall day. Protein requires the most work from your body to

break it down into its usable bits, and this is good news. Protein slows digestion, helping you to stay on point so you get lasting results.

- **Nourishment:** Proteins also contain B vitamins and minerals that help transform the food you eat into the health-giving nutrients, vitamins, and minerals your body needs to function all day long.

Since dietary proteins are the most demanding on your digestion regarding how they must be taken apart, you burn more calories digesting protein than any other nutrient.

When scientists talk about the rate at which you digest nutrients, they call it the thermic effect of food (TEF). The higher the demand on your digestion, the slower the TEF. When you eat protein, it requires you to use 25 to 30 percent of that protein's own energy just to digest itself, while carbs use a range from 5 to 30 percent depending on their complexity, and fats burn anywhere from 0 to 3 percent during digestion. In other words, protein takes the longest to digest.

Getting enough protein is how you keep your muscles from going to flab. Remember, eating protein is how your body's cells build protein. As you age, you need more protein to prevent muscle loss. Muscle helps you maintain a healthy weight and a toned body (and I'm not talking about big, bulky muscles) and gives you steady and long-lasting energy. According to a 2015 study from researchers who study aging and longevity, people who consumed twice as much protein as the current recommended daily average (RDA) found it easier to maintain and build muscle and had faster metabolisms than those who stuck with the RDA for protein.

During the eight-hour Boost Zone, you'll consume 20 percent of your calories from protein. This is the ideal amount of protein you'll need each day to get slim, trim, and toned. Remember, protein takes up much less space than stored fat does, so building muscle, which protein does, will make you smaller, not bigger or bulkier. Enough protein also curbs your appetite and reduces the risk of overweight, obesity, diabetes, and heart disease. I've got you covered. In the next chapter, you'll get your meal guide to the perfect amount of proteins. All you have to do is enjoy the delicious proteins included in the Four-Week Plan.

> **Quick Protein Tip:** I often carry Chomps jerky sticks with me for a fast protein snack without the guilt. They are the healthy version of Slim Jims and are made with 100 percent grass-fed and grass-finished beef, venison, or free-range antibiotic-free turkey, and are free of additives and preservatives. Not to mention they pack a punch with 9 to 10 grams of protein per stick with no added sugar, gluten, soy, or dairy. Hide these from your kids! My boys love them and if I leave them out, they are gone before I get even one (to buy, see Resources, page 303).

NAVIGATING PROTEINS

Sea-based proteins are best when wild-caught rather than farm-raised (the product packaging should indicate what's inside). Land-based proteins are best when grass-fed, free-range, unprocessed, and organic. I encourage you to use grass-fed and/or organic meats as often as possible. Vegetarian or vegan? Aim to get the right amount of protein from seeds, nuts, or a plant-based protein powder. If you eat eggs, choose those that are from pasture-raised and organic chickens.

Don't skimp on the fat! If you buy ground meat, go for the higher amounts of fat available. Choose 85 percent lean and 15 percent fat (or 80/20). Not only is animal fat good for your health, it's where all the flavor hides. Chicken and beef bone broth are also terrific protein sources. You may include turkey or beef bacon, as well as chicken, turkey, or beef sausage and hot dogs, but be sure to choose organic brands without added chemicals, carbs, sugars, or nitrates. I recommend avoiding pork and shellfish, since they can contain high levels of toxins.

Organic and/or grass-fed dairy is best. Cheeses from sheep's or goat's milk are easiest to digest. You can also have one tablespoon of grass-fed, organic cream and 4 ounces of organic cottage cheese each day.

Fats

I admit it's hard to get your head around the philosophy that jiggly, gelatinous, and greasy fat is good. And for goodness sakes, I get it. The muffin tops, arm jiggle, and back fat *are* made of fat, so why in the heck would you want to eat more of the stuff that's making it hard to squeeze into your skinny jeans? But the fat I'm talking about is different. Promise and cross my heart! Eating the fat on this meal plan will actually burn off that fatty excess on your body. You'll be consuming specific healthy fats that reduce chronically high insulin and anxiety, and improve your mood, slow your digestion (part of why you'll never feel ravenous), curb food cravings, keep your cells hydrated (which keeps your skin glowing), lower your cholesterol and blood sugar, and reduce the risk of all other disease and illness.

For more than five decades you've been taught that fat is the dastardly demon that causes heart attacks, clogged arteries, and obesity. So, despite the more recent promises you might have heard about fat, you may still feel resistant. It's a lot to swallow, especially after being repeatedly led down the dead end by following weight-loss promises that don't work. Here's the thing—while many have been taught that a low-fat diet is best, if you jump back a bit in time, you'll see that fat has been recommended for hundreds of years.

In the mid-1800s, a surgeon named Dr. William Harvey recommended a high-fat, low-carb plan to treat diabetes. Dr. Harvey suggested the diet to many, including a corpulent undertaker named William Banting. In 1863, after Banting's success with weight loss on this plan, he self-published a letter to the public with the rather lofty title: *Letter on Corpulence Addressed to the Public.* In it he detailed his success with Harvey's high-fat, low-carb guidelines. The letter went viral in the most old-fashioned way possible. It was turned into a printed pamphlet that was widely circulated in the late 1800s. It became so popular that "Banting" became a verb to describe eating in Harvey's prescribed way!

In the 1920s, doctors started using high-fat, low-carb diets to treat children with epilepsy, a treatment that is still used—with great success—today. In 1958, Dr. Richard Mackarness, author of *Eat Fat and Grow Slim,* promoted a low-carbohydrate meal plan that was similar to the Atkins diet (published in the '70s, but it didn't get attention until he updated it in the '90s), and then came hundreds of others such as the South Beach diet, the paleo diet, the Whole30 diet, the Primal Blueprint diet, and my own Belly Fat series. I'm not saying that these experts got *everything* right, but I still believe that they (we) were on the right track.

What does this tell us? That for hundreds of years, doctors, researchers, and other experts have known that fat can help your health—that it isn't dangerous or scary. Let's dive a little deeper into this topic.

What experts understand today that we lost sight of in the 1970s in the haze of the low-fat, high-carb craze is that *your body needs certain dietary fats to lose weight, to reduce the risk of heart disease, and to carry, absorb, and deliver nutrients throughout your body.* Fat also helps you to absorb vitamins better. And don't forget that most unprocessed, high-fat foods (think avocados and walnuts) are also crammed full with tons of nutrients, from vitamins and minerals to free-radical-fighting antioxidants.

Healthy fats burn more cleanly and contain more energy than carbs or proteins. Why? First of all, fats don't have to be put through any sort of metabolic assembly line to be stored or used in the body. Second, each gram of fat provides nearly twice as much energy as a gram of carbs or proteins.

The U.S. Dietary Guidelines and recommended daily levels miss the mark when they advocate less saturated fat and more polyunsaturated fats to lower the risk of heart disease. Just as all calories are not equally beneficial, neither are all fats. Let's put the pedal to the metal and take a closer look at high- versus low-octane fats.

STAN **CHEUNG**

AGE: 43 | WEIGHT LOST: 28 POUNDS

What everyone needs to know: Sweatpants don't have to be your daily uniform. If anyone had told me that just a few weeks before I'd started Cruise Control, I wouldn't have believed them.

I haven't worn jeans in fifteen years. I'm notorious for wearing sweats and workout pants. At. All. Times. Seriously.

Not only am I now wearing jeans, my wife told me that she didn't order them from the big and tall section. To top that, I tried on one of my biggest pants and I could fit both legs in one side. The other week I got lab results back from my doctor's visit and my blood sugar has dropped from diabetic to an entirely nondiabetic level! That's pretty unheard of for diabetics, and it's the result of which I'm most proud.

I once laughed at my extra weight and at myself by joining in a belly-flop competition on a cruise ship vacation (I won). Today, I Cruise every day, and I laugh in delight at my new and improved life on Cruise Control.

A FEW THINGS TO KEEP IN MIND ABOUT ALL FATS

All the fats you eat and all the fat that is stored in your body are triglycerides. Our doctors have taught us to fear these types of fats and with good reason. As a stored fat on your body, triglycerides can cause lots of health risks, including heart disease, diabetes, cancers, and general inflammation. However, it's important that you understand that when it comes to the chemical formation of fat—both in your body and in your food—it's always some variation on the same chemical equation: Three (tri-) fatty acids held together with glycerol (-glyceride) backbone. *In other words:* One glycerol backbone + (fatty acid + fatty acid + fatty acid) = a triglyceride. The chains of each of the fatty acids vary in length, some forming longer chains than others—and it's this difference that separates the good fats from the bad ones. Got it?

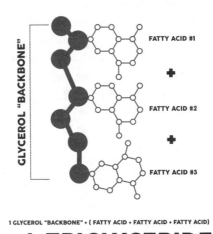

1 GLYCEROL "BACKBONE" + (FATTY ACID + FATTY ACID + FATTY ACID)

= A TRIGLYCERIDE

NAVIGATING FATS

THE GOOD FATS

The key thing about a *good* fat is that it comes to your plate or cup minimally to completely unprocessed. These fats can be quickly traced to their natural roots: avocados, nuts, eggs, seeds, certain fish, lean proteins, and healthy oils made from olives or walnuts. These good fats help your body burn the bad fatty tissues that are clogging and padding your body. Here are my favorites:

Stearic Acid
Where to find it: Cocoa butter, shea butter, milk, and butter
What it is: Long-chain saturated fat made of stearic acid
What's to love: The long length of these fatty acids keeps you feeling satisfied and full for longer. They therefore make an excellent appetite suppressant!

Lauric Acid
Where to find it: Coconut and palm kernel oil
What it is: Medium-chain saturated triglycerides (MCTs)
What's to love: Your body has a harder time making body fat from MCTs than it does from other types of dietary fat. That means that your body would rather burn this fat for energy than store it away as fat.

Oleic Acid
Where to find it: Olive oil, avocados, walnuts, grapeseed oil, macadamia nuts*
What it is: A monounsaturated omega-9 fatty acid.
What's to love: Oleic acid can help reduce appetite, improve energy, boost mood, and promote weight loss.
*A Note about Nuts and Seeds:** Unless otherwise noted, you'll want to keep nuts and seeds to ¼ cup or 1 ounce of nut or seed butter per day (2 tablespoons). Any of the nuts or seeds found on the Boost Zone list may be consumed raw or dry roasted. One easy way that I've learned to get my nuts is from a company called FBOMB. They come in pre-measured packets and have no added sugars or any of the bad fats that I want you to avoid (see "Drop an FBOMB," page 58, for more on this innovative and healthy way to get good fats in premeasured packages).

Eicosapentaenoic Acid (EPA) and Docosahexaenoic Acid (DHA)
Where to find it: Fish and algae supplements like spirulina
What it is: Omega-3 fatty acids found primarily in fish and algae supplements like spirulina
What's to love: These specific omega-3s are memory boosters, inflammation reducers, and belly-fat warriors! Some studies show that increased intake of these fats lowers your risk of Alzheimer's and heart disease.

Alpha-Linoleic Acid (ALA)
Where to find it: Flaxseeds, chia seeds, walnuts, kiwi, hemp, and grass-fed butter and beef
What it is: An omega-3 essential fatty acid, meaning it cannot be produced by the body
What's to love: This is a plant-based omega-3 that must be converted into the active forms of EPA and DHA after you've consumed it from food. Some research indicates that it may be more potent to get EPA and DHA directly from the seafood sources rather than having your body convert ALA into EPA and DHA. However, if you are vegan or vegetarian, this is a great option, and it comes with all the other benefits associated with these healthy fats.

Arachidonic Acid
Where to find it: Duck, chicken, halibut, wild salmon, eggs (yolks), beef
What it is: A polyunsaturated omega-6 fatty acid that is used by the body as a foundational starter kit to make other useful acids in your body
What's to love: This fat has been shown to improve the immune system and lean muscle while reducing inflammation. A recent review of AA found that it can improve mood and motivation and reduce stress.

Conjugated Linoleic Acid
Where to find it: Grass-fed beef, grass-fed dairy, and lamb
What it is: Naturally conjugated linoleic acids (CLAs) is the name given to a group of chemicals found in linoleic acid.
What's to love: Some research shows that this fat promotes the loss of body fat and weight.

DROP AN FBOMB

I love the power of real food, and I preach about not eating overly processed food that's full of chemicals and toxins. But I also really like it when food is there when I need it! Too bad it's so hard to find packaged food that doesn't have additives and preservatives and isn't overly processed. Enter FBOMB. Created by a couple named Kara and Ross Taylor, FBOMBs are handy packets of pure, healthy fats and nut butters. I wholeheartedly approve FBOMBs as Boost Zone snacks or as a replacement Boost Zone meal anytime.

FBOMB also makes packets of pure MCT oils and coconut oil, which makes for a perfect companion if you go on a long hike or to have after a workout. My bestie Brooke Burke, my in-laws, and I are all obsessed with these, and we carry them around with us for a fast snack or addition to our coffees. I love to bring these with me when I'm out at night or up early in the morning at a breakfast meeting. I can have a satisfying cup of Cruise Control Coffee or Tea (regular or decaf) by just dropping in a lil' ole FBOMB! For ordering information, see page 303.

THE BAD FATS

Man-made or synthetic fats are the absolute worst. These are the trans fats that are used in the making of movie popcorn "butter," candy bars, doughnuts, many store-bought cookies, and much, much more. Eating these fats is pretty much like eating plastic; it sort of *is* plastic to your body. Synthetic trans fats clog up your arteries like traffic in Los Angeles, they spike your bad cholesterol and smash your good cholesterol, and they'll also spike your risk of many diseases, including type 2 diabetes, heart disease, stroke, Alzheimer's, arthritis pain, cancer, and more. Here's the worst of the worst. Avoid these at all times!

Partially hydrogenated oils.
Where to find it: Fried and baked foods, margarine, and vegetable shortening

Linoleic acid.
Where you'll find it: Soybean oil, safflower oil, corn oil, poppy seed oil

Palmitic acid.
Where you'll find it: Palm oil, and animal fats from conventionally raised animals

The skinny on all this fat talk is that you've got to eat good fat to lose lousy fat.

During the eight-hour Boost Zone, you'll get about 50 percent of your calories from the healthiest fats, and in the sixteen-hour Burn Zone, you'll get 100 percent of your calories from the healthiest fats. You'll feel full and satisfied thanks to the naturally satiating ability that comes from it. Plus, you'll be switching out of the slow lane as you drop your sugar levels and teach your body to rely on healthy fat as a predominant fuel. That means you'll liberate stubborn stored fat from your body.

Carbs

Last but not least of the macronutrient triad are carbohydrates. The most basic of these come in the form of simple sugars such as glucose, sucrose, and fructose, which you'll find in refined whole grains and fresh fruit. Long chains of complex carbohydrates are in whole grains and veggies. I've already said a lot about carbohydrates when it comes to spiking insulin and causing your body to make and store fat, but that doesn't mean that they are all bad. Sure, it's pretty easy to see the glaring red-flag carbs from sugary drinks, Pringles, Wonder Bread, Frappuccinos, and Red Vines—these are zero-fiber foods that lay waste to your metabolism, your immune system, and most definitely your waist. But there *are* delicious, high-fiber, low-sugar carbs that I'll absolutely require you to eat on Cruise Control, and you'll get about 30 percent of your Boost Zone calories from carbs. Let's take a look.

Veggies: Veggies are complex carbs and are rich in phytonutrients, phytochemicals, vitamins, minerals, and antioxidants. They repair cell damage, are anti-inflammatory, reduce your risk of cancer, and naturally detoxify your body. These carbs are also gut-friendly and produce sugars and starches that nurture your gut microbiome.

Need more reasons to eat your veggies? How about the fact that vegetables fill your belly without padding it. They are low-calorie but high-fiber, which is the recipe you want when striving for weight loss. Fiber slows your digestion and scrubs out your insides. On the Cruise Control Diet, you'll be eating an abundance of the healthiest vegetables. The vegetables below appear in order from the most nutritious to those you'll use with caution.

High-Octane Veggies: Think leafy greens and cruciferous vegetables: broccoli, Brussels sprouts, cabbage, and cauliflower. These carbohydrates are high in fiber and water but low in calories and sugars. They are highly satisfying and won't spike your insulin or cause your body to store calories away as fat.

Low-Octane Veggies: Think tubers: sweet potatoes, yams, rutabagas, carrots, and beets. They sure are colorful (and that trait makes them helpful in supporting a healthy intestinal microbiome), and they provide vitamins and nutrients, but they also contain a good dose of sugar and should be consumed minimally.

Whole Grains: Think quinoa, brown rice, white rice, and air-popped popcorn. The general rule of thumb for this category is that they are somewhat to completely unprocessed grains. As such, they contain the fiber and nutrients that will help you have regular bowel movements, and have been linked to reducing inflammation and cancer risk.

Starch: Avoid potatoes, corn, and refined flours. These are carbs that spike your blood sugar and trigger your insulin. They are high in starch and low in fiber, which means your body processes them just like sugar and they end up stored as fat on your body. This isn't to say that you will entirely ban these carbohydrates, but you will want to minimize them. One of the problems with striking all starch from your diet is that it can affect your mood. Your body wants at least a little of this fuel. The important thing to remember is to stick to the most colorful low-octane starches, such as sweet potatoes and yams, and avoid the bland colored ones. Thankfully, I've found some really great subs for pasta, such as the one made by Palmini, which is a pasta made with hearts of palm that tastes amazingly like the real stuff (see "My Secret Pasta Swap," below).

Fruits: Here's the deal with Mother Nature's dessert—have fruit as a treat once or twice a week, or once or twice a day if your body permits it, but no more. Once upon a time, we humans could safely gorge on a field of blackberries because we didn't have them handy twenty-four hours a day, seven days a week. Thanks to the fact that most of us have been conditioned to eating a diet that causes elevated levels of insulin (too many simple and refined carbs), fruit has become something that we need to enjoy sparingly. Your best bets are berries of any type, and you'll see these incorporated into Cruise Control.

MY SECRET PASTA SWAP

Okay, so not everyone is a fan of spiralizing their own veggies or of the texture or carb counts of brown rice pastas. Now there's an alternative! I recently discovered Palmini Pasta, a product that's made from healthy hearts of palm, and tastes remarkably like real pasta. You might have found this where I did, watching an episode of *Shark Tank*. It makes a fast dinner thanks to just needing a quick zap in the microwave or heating on your stovetop. And hey, if my middle-schooler eats it and thinks it's the real thing, then end of story, am I right? You can find these in Whole Foods stores and on Amazon.com.

Palmini Pasta has only 4 grams of carbs and just 20 calories per serving! It's a great substitute you can use in the Zoodle Spaghetti & Meatballs recipe found on page 171 (for more information, see Resources, page 307).

Fruit that comes in cans or jars is prohibited on Cruise Control, but fresh or frozen fruit is allowed. Choose local *and* organic whenever possible. Enjoy two pieces or servings of any of the low-sugar fruits found on the Boost Zone list (see page 135). Fruit can be eaten as a snack in between lunch and dinner, with meals, or as an after-dinner treat. Enjoy fresh lemon and lime juice as a great addition to your water anytime (you don't have to count lemon or lime juice in water as part of your daily fruit allotment).

Artificial Sweeteners

I don't recommend artificial sweeteners. The only sweeteners that I do approve of are monk fruit, stevia, xylitol, and erythritol. Artificial and other sugar-free sweeteners fool your body into thinking they are sugar, causing it to release insulin, which causes it to store fat. Monk fruit, stevia, xylitol, and erythritol are natural and do not have this effect if used in moderation. Make sure to consume pure stevia, erythritol, or monk fruit extracts with no sugars or starches added. Read labels carefully and stick to those sweeteners found on my approved food lists (see page 130)! You want to avoid any product that lists sugar or artificial sweeteners as ingredients. Don't know what some of those words mean? I'll help you here: stay away from fructose, sucrose, acesulfame potassium, aspartame, saccharin, and sucralose. That means no pink, blue, or yellow packets! More places are starting to carry stevia, but I always like to have some packets of Swerve sweetener or stevia in my bag just to be sure.

ELGHA **DILWORTH**

AGE: 60 | WEIGHT LOST: 10 POUNDS

What everyone needs to know: You'll be able to stop hiding. I have firmed up so much in the last few weeks that I was able to go to yoga for the first time in ten years without wearing a big baggy top to hide all my bits—and I felt, and looked, great.

MY GO-TO SWEETENER

It's hard to find a replacement for sugar that doesn't hurt your health or one that doesn't come with a funky aftertaste. I really like Swerve because you can bake with it as well as use it in cold beverages and plain yogurts. But that's not all! Swerve sells several different kinds of sweetener, including confectioners' sugar replacement for frosting, brown sugar replacement, cake and cookie mixes, and pancake and waffle mix. Swerve is zero-calorie, it's made from fruits and starchy root vegetables, but it won't spike your blood sugar or signal your insulin, so it's safe to use in your Boost or your Burn Zones. Swerve baking sugar works perfectly in my decadent recipe Chocolate Salted Peanut Butter Cups, which you can find on page 189. It's delicious! For more information, see Resources, page 306.

Fermented Foods

Eat fermented foods such as sauerkraut, kimchi, assorted fermented veggies, raw apple cider vinegar (ACV), and raw coconut vinegar. These foods promote a healthy gut environment, improve digestion, boost immunity, and can help you to maintain a healthy weight.

Seasonings and Herbs

Seasonings and herbs offer great flavoring options for your meals, especially if you are a picky eater. Plus, they are jam-packed with antioxidants! Enjoy fresh or dry herbs and spices liberally but take a moment to check labels. You don't want any added monosodium glutamate (MSG), glutamic acid, sugar, dextrose, or natural sweeteners. Some of my favorite approved seasonings and herbs include vinegar, basil, garlic powder, hot peppers, oregano, and thyme. These can really spice up the flavor and complexity of vegetables. Check the list on page 129 and recipes for more.

Beverages

The biggest rule when it comes to beverages is to avoid any drink that has added sugar or artificial sweeteners. Got that? Nothing with added sugar or artificial sweeteners! Need a little flavor in your water? Try lemon juice, orange juice, grapefruit juice, peppermint, or even cinnamon. You can also enjoy a splash of unsweetened almond or coconut milk in your coffee and teas or herbal infusions any time of the day.

Let's take a quick but closer look at water—it's that important; there's just no better drink. What's so great about H_2O? Water hydrates your cells, and cellular hydration is a critical part of fat burning. If your cells are dehydrated, oxygen and essential nutrients can't get inside. This can cause a toxic buildup of metabolic waste. If your cells aren't firing on all pistons, your body's engine can't perform optimally. Hydration is also necessary for cells to make energy. That's why you feel fatigued when you don't drink enough water. Hydrated cells trigger many mechanisms in the body that help it to release the right hormones in the right amounts, and to synthesize proteins. Hydrated cells are better able to reduce acidity, and to increase fat burning, DNA repair, and immunity. The other thing to remember is that the feeling of hunger can often be thirst. So before you eat something, drink a glass of water. If your hunger abates, it means that you were really just thirsty. I recommend purified water whenever possible.

How much, you ask? Aim to get around half your body weight in ounces for the best health benefits.

FREELY

WATER

COFFEE

TEA

OTHER RULES TO DRINK BY?

MODERATELY

ALMOND

MILK

WINE

- You can drink up to three coffees or caffeinated teas per day before 2:00 P.M. Caffeine later in the afternoon can disrupt sleep.
- Herbal and decaffeinated teas can be enjoyed anytime.
- Milk should also be used in moderation because it has its own sugars.

RARELY

SPIRITS

- If you drink milk—almond, coconut, soy, or dairy—make sure that it is unsweetened.

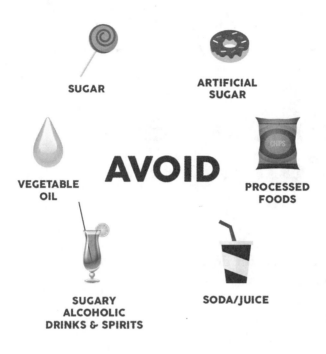

IN CASE IT WASN'T CLEAR . . .

Eating the wrong foods will cause your arteries to harden and clog up (think French fries and chips), which increases your risk of high blood pressure and heart disease, and many other health issues. Also, unhealthy foods make your thinking foggy, cause poor concentration, and make you look older than your years. This is why you wake up all puffy, with bags under your eyes, the night after you indulge in a pizza with the works. Refined carbs and sugary foods are addictive. Research shows that they trigger the same parts of the brain as cocaine and other highly addictive drugs. That's why you repeatedly crave and binge on these "foods." Chips and candy bars beget more chips and candy bars. Finally, highly processed, refined, and sugary products hurt your digestive system and have been linked to heart disease, cancer, diabetes, and more.

CHAPTER 4

Mindset & Motivation

> There is a powerful driving force inside every human being that, once unleashed, can make any vision, dream, or desire a reality.
> —TONY ROBBINS

Cruise Control is a lifestyle, but it only works if you keep your head in the game. As we've discussed, there's no special product, procedure, regimen, or equipment you need—except your own mind. That's right. Your conscious intention is the greatest driving force available to you when it comes to making your dreams and desires a reality. You won't be on Cruise Control, you'll be *living* Cruise Control, and to really live requires self-examination, self-reflection, mindfulness, conscious intention, positive thinking, and empowered self-love. I want you to be genuinely awake to your reality each and every day. You need your mind on board to follow the route that will take you to ultimate success, health, and happiness.

You know the fundamentals of Cruise Control. Now it's time to upload your navigation center. Your mind is like Google Maps: it can help you get to where you want to go, but only if it is given the correct information. If you fill it with a bunch of junk—negative, closed, and rigid thinking—it can and will steer you wrong. Here is where you're going to get the brain algorithms and a few practical strategies that will give you the final turbocharge to keep you on track toward your goals. In this chapter, you'll learn how to boost your success, set achievable goals, be mindful about tracking and check-ins, engage in empowered self-talk, and navigate mind blocks.

In the last part of this chapter, we'll review common mind blocks. You'll learn how to drive around, over, or through any obstacles on the road to your dream destination—health, happiness, and vitality. These powerful mindful strategies for creating your own empowering mantras, mind maps, journaling, and other tools will keep you motivated and revved up for an *extremely* long, healthy, and happy life.

COMMITMENT IS THE KEY TO SUCCESS

Devotion, loyalty, tenacity, grit—above anything else, your success depends on your own internal willingness and motivation to commit to the importance and priority of owning your own health. You must set your own intention. As Louise Hay, the master of healing oneself, always told me, "Claim it!" No one else will ever care about your health more than you. Despite complete confidence in Cruise Control, I still know it won't work unless you are ready to claim what you deserve, your *best* health and life.

While I know that you'll see fast results on Cruise Control, your success hinges on your ability to see this as a cross-country road trip, not a 60-meter foot race. Commitment isn't a one-time thing; you must continue to renew your body and mind every single day. You must challenge your old thoughts and beliefs and replace them with new opinions and aspirations. So are you ready to ditch that old clunker of a body and brain, and upgrade to the latest model of health? I've discovered five commitments that, when internalized and implemented, will guarantee your success.

THE 5 COMMITMENTS

1. **Pledge to the process, not a product:** It would be nice if there were "magic bullet" products or a procedure that would zap us all into instant health and flawless beauty, but let's get real. You know as well as I do that real change *really* happens when you put in the effort, and lasting change doesn't often happen overnight. Commit to this transformative process that combines nutrition, movement, and accountability.

2. **Commit to a lifestyle, not a diet:** Dieting doesn't work. We've been beaten over the head with research that proves this point. When you adopt the long-term healthy lifestyle that is Cruise Control, you won't ever feel the deprivation, restriction, cravings, or binges that go hand in hand with diets. Your lifestyle is simply the style of your life. It's something you can live with long-term. Cruise Control won't trend in or out like bell-bottom pants or platform shoes—or diets. A lifestyle is what it sounds like, enjoyable and vibrant. The *side* benefits are that excess fat melts off your body, your mind wakes up, and you are energized with life's highest-octane fuel.

3. **Own positivity, ditch negativity:** Most people beat themselves up over occasional slipups. Research in the field of psychology proves that focusing on your wins and what you're doing right creates long-term transformation. The Cruise Control program is designed to provide rapid results and daily "victories" that you can celebrate.

4. **Be the driver, not the driven:** You will never create happiness and long-term change if you don't take responsibility for your situation. It might be true that you were handed some fat genes, or that you were raised in a family of fast-food addicts, but today you choose. Cruise Control puts you in the driver's seat; no one will ever chauffeur you to bad health (or bad food) again.

5. **Belong, don't be alone:** Research shows that your weight, income, and happiness are directly tied to the people in your community. Do you hang with heavy drinkers, eaters, or sofa slugs? Or do you consider yourself an island of isolation? Neither extreme is ideal. Remember number four above: you are the driver of your life. That means that you have the power to surround yourself with healthy,

loving people—not energy vampires or negative, judgmental types. People in recovery have a saying: "If you hang around a barbershop, you are probably going to get a haircut." It's the same when you are "recovering" from an unhealthy lifestyle. If you hang around the open bar at a wedding, or if you frequent an all-you-can-eat buffet regularly, you'll probably drink and eat more than is beneficial. No more! There's a Cruise Control family that is waiting to welcome and support you. Visit www.jorgecruise.com, and start hanging with the winners.

WHAT TO EXPECT

Yes, you can drop up to twenty-eight pounds in the first four weeks on Cruise Control, but understand that not all of that weight will come directly from fat. More likely, 10 to 15 percent of the weight you lose will be fat, but much of the rest of it will come from inflammation-related water retention. Think of inflammation in your body as a fire in a part of a house. Your body tries to keep water where there is inflammation to "cool" the fire in that part of the "house." When you start eating the Cruise Control way, you'll reduce inflammation, and you'll let go of that water.

The other source of weight loss that you'll see is what I refer to as "false fat," which is simply trapped waste matter in your body. I know it is unpleasant to imagine this buildup in your body, but the good news is that you're about to flush the junk out of your system rapidly. You'll see a lot of this in the first week. And regardless of where this weight loss comes from, you're going to look slimmer—fast! A lot of what gives you that bloated stomach discomfort is a buildup of waste in your intestines, the result of eating all day long. You'll give your body the break it needs during your daily Burn Zone, effectively revving up your digestive system and helping your body clean out your pipes. You'll also get plenty of fiber during your Boost Zone that comes from Cruise Control carbs. Fiber is another essential component that your body needs to remove rubbish from it; eating a diet of highly refined, processed carbs and sugars clogs up your intestines with sewage. No matter how much you have to lose, your results will be dramatic, and you will look and feel fantastic and renewed. Take a look at what to expect each week:

YOUR GOAL TOTAL	EACH WEEK
Lose 60+ pounds	7 to 10 pounds
Lose 40 to 60 pounds	6 to 9 pounds
Lose 20 to 40 pounds	5 to 8 pounds
Lose 10 to 20 pounds	3 to 5 pounds
Lose 3 to 10 pounds	1 to 3 pounds

SUCCESS BOOSTERS: GOAL PLANNING FOR SUCCESS (GPS)

Having goals is a fundamental component of success because they give you the ability to visualize a version of the future you desire—goals fuel motivation. But there's more to knowing your desired target than just saying or writing it as if you were making a wish list for Santa. Goal success relies on your beliefs, your desire, your deep *want* for an identified wish to come true. You must be fully invested, and to do that requires contemplation and commitment. Setting goals will help you grow and expand, but only if you include some essential steps and strategies. If I want to go on a road trip with my family to see Yellowstone Park, I don't just hop in my car and start driving, and, as nice as it would be, it doesn't just magically happen if I tell my husband I want to go. We need to consider our route, and I know I'll have a much better time if I do some research ahead of time and prioritize what I really want to see when we get there.

Going on a road trip isn't free, and neither is Cruise Control. Everything comes with a cost, but in both cases, the extra work will be worth it, and the payoff is amazing! You'll be less likely to get lost or get stuck, sidelined by detours or other obstacles. To push yourself to transform your body and life successfully takes thoughtful planning. Don't worry. This part is fun. Taking the time to visualize the life of your dreams, to grab hold with tenacity and grit to what you've always wished you could have—this is what it takes to reach your goals. This is how you get to that "powerful driving force" inside yourself. By the time you're done with setting your goals, you'll wake up each morning revved to go fast. Think of it as a dream with a deadline. Let's look a little deeper at why your motives and reasons come first, how to identify them, and then how to set your goals. First, grab a pen and a spiral notebook or journal.

Reasons First, Results Second: I always say reasons come first, results come second. You might know that you want to lose twenty pounds, but have you taken the time to think about why? It's important to understand the reasons behind your goals—this is where the true motivation lies. For example, "I want to lose twenty pounds so that I can go camping with my grandkids this summer" is a goal that has a meaningful reason behind it. The more descriptive you can be about your reasons for wanting your goal, the more you strengthen your intention and ability to reach it.

1. Determine your goals: What do you want? I want you to set three goals for yourself while doing Cruise Control. Go ahead. Don't hold back. Have that pen and paper? Jot down a list of what you want. Scientific research shows that you'll be more than 40 percent as likely to reach your goals and dreams when you write them down, versus just thinking about them. Why? Your brain is divided into two hemispheres. The right side of your brain is where your imagination lives; the left is where logical thinking happens. You need both sides of your brain to communicate to make a goal you've imagined into a reality, and when you pick up a pen or pencil and write something down, it sends a signal from both sides of your brain and brings it all together. The message your entire being then gets is committed and inspired—"I am going to get to this goal"—in every cell in your body!

So, grab your paper and your pen. Set your timer for five minutes and brainstorm a list of anything you'd like to achieve, create, do, have, give, and/or experience in the next four weeks. Write as many things down as fast as you can in this time. There are no rules. Your goals can be anything you want them to be, but only one is about weight loss. Focus your other two on non-scale victories, like fitting into those skinny jeans you have or getting off blood pressure medications. Have fun and really think about what you want Cruise Control to do for you—the possibilities are endless! When you are done, go back and circle the three things that are the most important to you. Here are some examples of non-weight-related goals:

- I want to be more patient and less irritable.
- I want to feel serene and tranquil.
- I want to feel energized all day long.
- I want to be stronger.
- I want to have more flexibility.
- I want my back and neck to stop hurting.
- I want to sleep better.
- I want to stop eating junk food, sugar, etc.
- I want to climb Machu Picchu.
- I want to live to see my kids grow up.
- I want to have more self-confidence.

2. Investigate your motivation: On a clean sheet of paper, rewrite your three goals, leaving space between each one. Now, why do you want these things? What will they bring you? Remember, it's the act of writing that brings ultimate brain power by signaling and empowering both the creative and the logical sides of your brain.

Now write out your intention, explaining why you are absolutely 100 percent motivated to achieve these goals within the next four weeks. Get as specific as you can. Look at your first goal. Think about why it's important to you. What are the personal "reasons" behind the goal? For example: "I want to lose twenty pounds so that I am no longer out of breath when I walk up the stairs in my home." Go deeper. Why do you want to not be out of breath? Maybe you hate the tight feeling in your chest, or perhaps you feel embarrassed when others see you huffing and puffing.

3. Review weekly: Go to your calendar (whether electronic or on paper) and put in a goal-review reminder for each week of the next four weeks. Also, ask a friend to remind you to review your goals once a week. The more you repeat your goals, the more your brain will get the message that this is important information that must be remembered. If you keep these on your phone, you can have an alert that will pop up every seven days, but I still want you to write about your goals and talk about them. You can also take a picture of your goals and save them as the background on your laptop or phone.

STRATEGIES TO MOTIVATE AND WIN

Being prepared with the following exercises and tools will keep your mind *cruising* forward, so you stay revved up and motivated to reach your goals. Read on for my favorites. These tips keep countless clients and me moving forward even when we hit life's roadblocks, obstacles, and detours:

Create and Use Affirmations: Your Thoughts Become Your Actions

Louise Hay, the late publisher and author—most famously of *You Can Heal Your Life*—was the first person to take a chance on me as an author, and I think of her as the mother of positive thinking and the law of attraction. She taught me that if you aren't happy with your life, you first need to start to make changes in your mind. Just because you've believed something for a long time doesn't mean you have to accept it as a truth forever. You can change the thoughts you have about yourself, and when you do, you can change your life. The key to doing this is to create space between you and whatever thought you have—and the way to create this space is to use affirmations.

An affirmation is a phrase that you repeat, either out loud or silently to yourself, to verbalize and visualize what you want in your life. I started using affirmations in 2005, when Louise told me that what you say to yourself mentally is powerful, and if you believe it you can become it. This can work for you and against you. If you allow a negative thought to persist, it can take over your life and inform your actions, or inaction.

You tell yourself you aren't good enough or that you'll never be able to change. It's a negative tape that plays all day long. "I can't lose weight, I'm too fat, I hate my belly." These are negative declarations, and they reinforce negative beliefs. Replacing this negative self-talk with positive statements stops negative thinking like a red light, and turns it to green so you can move forward with new positive beliefs.

Going from a self-destructive mindset to a positive frame of reference and self-love won't happen instantaneously. However, I can assure you that if you practice these affirmations over time, you'll start to notice your thinking changes. The key is to keep them positive and to say them as if they are a reality that is already happening in your life. You can write your own, or use one of the following:

- I love myself just as I am.
- *In the morning:* I have power and wisdom to have a fantastic day.
- *In the evening:* I did a great job today; I love myself, and I'm proud of my success.
- I flow with life easily and effortlessly.
- I love foods that energize my body and soul.
- I am letting go of past fears about food; I will eat to live, I will not live to eat.
- I make choices and decisions for my best health.
- I am repairing, rejuvenating, and reinvigorating my life.
- I celebrate myself and the positive food choices I make today.
- I accept my body for the shape I have been blessed with.
- I let go of relationships that are no longer beneficial to my health.
- I happily embrace new lessons in life.
- I take the time to be silent and count all the things for which I am grateful.
- I am a valuable person who deserves love and respect.
- My feelings are valid and deserve to be felt.
- I am grateful for my body and all it does for me every day.
- I am closer and closer to my ideal weight with each and every day.
- My beliefs and actions are in harmony with my goals.
- I accept my body exactly the way it is, and I continually work on improving it.

- I am losing weight, and nothing stands in the way of the body of my dreams.
- I am a magnificent and radiant being.

"But Jorge, what if I just don't believe it?" It's a question I get from clients all the time when I tell them to start looking in the mirror and say, "I am beautiful just as I am." As much as you ultimately want to believe what you are saying, affirmations give you a starting point. I think of these positive phrases as a way of planting seeds for a positive mindset. You might not see a sprout today, but keep nourishing that seed with good thoughts, and pretty soon you'll have a beautiful flower.

Design a Vision Board

Gather up a bunch of old magazines, maybe some favorite pictures, and get some colored pens and a poster board. Don't forget the glue or tape.

- Find pictures that show the goals you will reach. This might be a picture of someone on a Jet Ski, or a person running a marathon, or maybe it's a picture of the body you will have.
- Inspiring words: Include words like "peaceful" or "energized" or "relaxed." Reading words like this will help your brain make them a reality.
- Include pictures that show how you'll feel when you reach your goal.
- Cut out pictures of books that are inspiring to you.
- Include favorite quotes.
- Take a picture of you with your support group—your "carpool"—and put it on your collage.
- Include pictures of anything you love that expresses joy and bliss to you, such as butterflies, hummingbirds, flowers, etc.

Drive a Mindful Kitchen

Let's face it, your kitchen is your own personal food delivery system. You can either have a fridge and cupboards filled with junk foods or healthful foods—it's up to you. What does this have to do with staying motivated? Everything. Remember, visual cues are potent cues. That's why it's much easier to stay away from sugary and highly processed foods if you don't have to *see* them on your shelves. So, step one, clean out the crap. Take inventory of what you have. Look in your cupboards, refrigerator, and definitely in that place where you keep your secret stash of snacks. If you aren't willing to ditch anything, at least designate one hard-to-reach area for any foods that are a weakness. Way up above the fridge maybe? Or in a basement freezer. If you need to, inform those in your house where you have moved these foods, so they are not constantly asking where the chips and cookies have gone.

Create an Emotionally Nourishing Eating Area

It doesn't just stop in your kitchen. Creating a social and serene space where you can eat will help you to notice the fuel you're putting into your body. You'll be relaxed and eat more slowly (better for your digestion), and you won't overeat. This doesn't have to be in a formal dining room, but I do suggest that you sit in an area that feels peaceful and beautiful. This can be on your patio, on your deck, in a park, or even in another room of your house, as long as it isn't in front of any sort of screen. Also, when you eat in a social setting, it's important to have ground rules. No politics, no religion, and no upsetting conversation. You don't want to associate anything negative with your eating times.

Keep a Daily Motivation Tracker

Every day you should review your motivation. A checklist could work, but I don't want this part of the program to be too automatic. It's important to be engaged in your journey, to self-reflect on your progress, and to see if you need to make any adjustments. The best way to do this is in a notebook or journal. I like to do it each morning before I start my day. I take a minute to think about yesterday. How did it go? Did I follow my intended path? How did I feel? Could I have done anything better? And don't forget to include something that you accomplished, a success, as well as those things for which you are grateful. Gratitude is greatness and noting it is a well-known motivator. Then turn your attention to the day ahead of you. What's on your to-do list? What are your motives? What can wait until tomorrow? How will you care for yourself today?

You can close by writing out a favorite affirmation, or create a new one. Each new day, review what you wrote the day before. I also keep a gratitude journal that I write in on a daily basis. It's hard to be stressed or scared when you are grateful for all the blessings in your life.

Rally Your Support System

I want you to identify three people in your life whom you can count on as your own personal high-performance pit crew. This can be especially helpful when it comes to emotional eating. It's a lonely job, losing weight—it might be your own personal race to better health—but that doesn't mean you need to do it alone, and you shouldn't. We all need and deserve support. Instead of turning to food for comfort, you will turn to your Cruise Control crew: friends and family you can rely upon. After you've decided on your trio of teammates, ask one person to be your email or text buddy, one whom you can talk to in person or on the phone, and a third person who is willing to call you once a week to check in with you on how you are doing. By establishing your own personal Cruiser crew of support, you'll cut down on the risk and cost that comes from doing things alone, and you'll increase the likelihood of your success. This team can include family members, coworkers, and good friends—anyone you feel comfortable talking with openly and honestly. Choose teammates who are nonjudgmental, willing to listen, and supportive. It's important to make sure that your accountability buddy is someone you admire and strive to be like. If you have trouble finding a support system, join my community of Cruisers who are already having a blast on their weight loss and health journeys. Check in with other people going through the program by using #CruiseControlDiet and #JorgeCruise on Instagram and Facebook. This will help you stay accountable and get support from other community members. We're excited to see your progress!

Driving through Mind Blocks

It's easy to become overwhelmed, especially when starting a new lifestyle, but I want you to begin this journey on Cruise Control knowing that there are no mistakes. Obstacles, issues, circumstances, and roadblocks? Yeah. Those are going to happen. But here's the thing: each time you see a rock in your road, you have an opportunity to learn and grow, even if it goes wrong—even if it's horrible. You get in the wrong marriage or relationship, accept the wrong job, miss a deadline, eat a sleeve of Oreos—it's all part of the twists and turns, the hills and valleys—the full catastrophe (good and bad) of any journey. Your losses can wake you up and show you a better or wiser way to live. I was devastated when my mom died. I thought it was the most horrible thing to have ever happened to me, but today I know that I've grown and evolved in ways that I wouldn't have if I hadn't lost my mom, and I'm so grateful to have had her in my life for as long as I did. It doesn't erase the sadness, but that experience did show me that I could take the most horrible tragedy in my past and use it to help others and to help myself. When I am working with clients who have experienced the loss of someone they love, I can connect with them in a way that I couldn't before I lost my mom. I have a deeper understanding and compassion that the younger Jorge didn't have.

So relax, it's going to be okay—I've got your back. And even if you feel like you've been on a detour for a long time, you have the power at any moment you choose to use your experience to move in a new direction. Don't let yourself be thrown off course, just reroute and get better directions. That is the key.

So how do you get back on track when you have a rough day? The way through the challenge is to get still, pause, wait. It might feel like you are doing nothing, but waiting is actually a remarkably powerful action. When you are caught up in the midst of *any* erratic emotion, you can't use the part of your brain that helps you to problem solve. You revert back to using your old reptile brain and can only react. Let the ripples settle. Breathe. When you are calm, ask yourself what the next right move might be. If that doesn't do the trick, daily meditation can also be extremely helpful; see chapter 9, page 259, for more emotion-stabilizing tips.

While following the Cruise Control Diet, you may encounter challenges. Here are some tips, categorized by topic, to help you stay on track.

Staying Motivated When Emotions Come Calling: Emotional Eating

"Starve the emptiness and feed the hunger," sing the Indigo Girls. It's one of my favorite lyrics because it nails how emotional eating works. So many of us have been taught that food is love, a cure for boredom, or a way to tamp down stress and anger. When you try to fill emotional holes with food, the only thing you fill up is your belly (and butt and thighs). Your appetite will decrease, and hunger will be satisfied on Cruise Control, but that won't stop emotional triggers for eating. The next time you experience an emotional eating trigger, try the following:

Identify the Emotion: When you want to eat, but you know you aren't hungry, pause and identify what you are feeling. Understanding the underlying emotions that you associate with a desire to eat is the first step to freeing yourself from an unhealthy relationship with food.

Feel Your Feelings: This is the least fun tip in the whole book, but it's also possibly the most important. Feelings are great when we're talking about happiness and love, but not so much when you are feeling angry, sad, anxious, or bored. The good news is that feelings ebb and flow, even if it feels like they are never going to end, and the best way to deal with your feelings is to *feel* them. It's okay. They won't last. They aren't facts.

Call Someone: Don't text, don't email, and don't stew in isolation. If you can't calm down, talk to a trusted friend on the phone or in person.

Move: Move your body, move your mind. Take a walk, jog in place, do some yoga. Any sort of movement is a fantastic outlet for unpleasant feelings.

Shut Down: This doesn't sound like a healthy tip, but sometimes, if you just need to calm whatever fires are roaring in your head, it can help to watch a movie, binge on a show, or snuggle up and read a book. Taking a bath and a nap are good ideas, too. I'm not suggesting that you do this for days on end, but every now and then you might need some time to hit the reset button, and that's just fine.

TRACK YOUR MILEAGE

The following practices will help you stay motivated and moving forward on the road to success.

Picture Your Progress!

Many Cruisers begin to see results and changes in as little as three days, so imagine the transformation that can take place in twenty-eight! Document this exciting time—take photos. A few tips:

Wear Fitted Clothing: This goes for both your "before" and "after" photos. You want to be sure to see your entire shape.

Wear the Same Clothing in Each Photo: When you get to the finish line on day twenty-eight, make sure you take at least one picture in the same outfit you wore in your "before" photos. You'll be amazed at how much bigger those clothes look and feel.

No Selfies: Ask a friend or partner to take your photos. It may be tempting to take a selfie or try to capture a quick shot in the mirror, but you'll get a better result by having someone else take a full-body shot at a distance.

Go Natural and High-Def: Be sure to stand in a well-lighted, shadow-free setting, so you don't hide any subtle transformations. High dynamic range (HDR on most phones) lets you compare all the nuances of your transformation. If you're willing, I'd love it if you shared your progress on social media. Just hashtag #CruiseControlDiet and #JorgeCruise.

Capture Every Angle: Make sure to take photos from the front, back, and sides. You want a 360-degree view of your body before and after Cruise Control.

Weigh Yourself Weekly: I always recommend weighing yourself on the same day, once a week, in the morning, immediately after you get out of bed and use the bathroom. This will help ensure consistency in measurements. Some people prefer to weigh themselves daily, but I find that the majority of my clients who do this get discouraged because weight can fluctuate from day to day and you'll get more reliable results from weekly weigh-ins.

Measure Your Middle: Many of you will start seeing the inches come off in as little as three days, and since belly fat melts first on Cruise Control, you'll especially want to know your waist-to-hip ratio. A healthy waist-to-hip ratio for women is 0.7, and for men, it's 1.0.

To Take this Measurement: Take a fabric tape measure and, while sucking in your belly, measure your waist at the level of your belly button. Next, measure your hips at the largest point around your bottom. Finally, divide your waist size by your hip size. For example, if you have hips that are 46 inches and a waist that is 40 inches, then your waist-to-hip ratio is 0.86. Write all three measurements down—waist, hips, and waist-to-hip. You can remeasure every three to four days. Seeing the inches melt off your body is a great way to stay motivated.

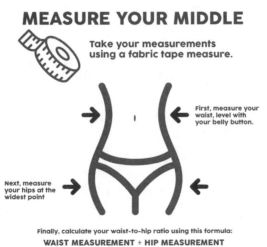

MEASURE YOUR MIDDLE

Take your measurements using a fabric tape measure.

First, measure your waist, level with your belly button.

Next, measure your hips at the widest point

Finally, calculate your waist-to-hip ratio using this formula:
WAIST MEASUREMENT ÷ HIP MEASUREMENT = WAIST-TO-HIP RATIO

Own It! Put Yourself First: Oprah Winfrey once explained to me that you have to fill yourself up first before you can give anything to anyone else. It's so easy for us to put our family, job, friends, and household first. The problem is that if you don't take care of yourself, you ultimately won't be any good to anyone else. It isn't selfish, it's self-care. Simply put: I want you to put yourself at the very top of your priority list for the next twenty-eight days.

Don't get me wrong. I'm not suggesting that you quit your job, fire your friends, or walk out on your family, but I am telling you to make yourself number one. Nurture yourself, honor yourself, and shut down the constant and negative self-defeating mental chatter that's going on in your head. Be good to yourself.

You've given so much. Now it is time for you to do some self-care and improve your health. I want you to sign a contract not only with yourself but with me, and the millions of Cruisers like you who are getting in the driver's seat to their best health. Use the following contract as a template. Rewrite it by hand or on your laptop (print it), sign it in ink, hang it where you can see it, and take a picture of it. Post it on my social media, #CruiseControlDiet. I promise I'll like it and comment back!

I, _____, commit to following Cruise Control for the next four weeks because I am worth it. I am fully committed to my health and body.

My Motivation is _____

_____

Signature _____

Date_____

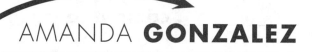

AMANDA **GONZALEZ**

AGE: 42 | WEIGHT LOST: 50 POUNDS

What everyone needs to know: It only took me one day to become a Cruiser! Not to say that I didn't have my reservations. At first, I was afraid. I love bread and sugar, and I didn't see any on Cruise Control. Still, I had spent the last year and a half eating poorly or trying to starve myself, but I just kept gaining weight. I was having difficulty sleeping at night. I had two babies just thirteen months apart, and both were born with severe defects that required surgery, and still, my youngest will have severe struggles her whole life. I got depressed and felt like I wanted to give up. When I read about Cruise Control, it gave me a glimmer of hope. I realized that it wasn't just about me anymore. My kids needed me. Maybe this Burning and Boosting could help me? I'd packed on more than fifty pounds. It sounded easy enough, eat for eight hours and have approved drinks and treats during the other sixteen. I decided to try it for one day, and then I'd see how I felt. Thanks to the Burn Zone treats, it was easy, and I really liked having chocolate and wine as a treat in the evening; that helped me not miss the bread and sugar I'd been so used to having.

I believe that it's up to us to decide if we are going to let the pain of life's circumstances take us down, or if we will develop and come out even more beautiful than before. It's taken me forty-two years to realize that I need to value what I put in my body. We all have things in our lives that can break us. I once read that a pearl can take five to twenty years to develop inside an oyster. Think of yourself as a pearl, be patient, and give yourself the time you need to grow and become beautiful.

CHAPTER 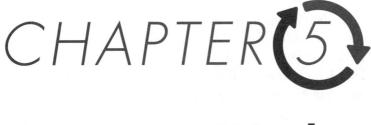 5

Your Four-Week Plan

The greatest wealth is health.
—VIRGIL

Y ou know how Cruise Control works, the benefits you can expect, and the nutrition logic that is behind the design of this effortless drive-through lifestyle. You are now ready to begin your new life on Cruise Control and to claim effortless fat-burning and total health forever. In this chapter, we'll start with the five commitments that you'll make to guarantee your success on Cruise Control. Then you'll get going on the "how it works" portion of the plan. This includes your meal planners, shopping lists, and approved Cruise Control food lists to Boost and Burn. I've designed all of this to be as simple and automated as possible. At the end of the chapter, you'll learn how to transition after your four weeks into your fifth week, and all the weeks beyond.

Your transformation begins today!

CHOOSE YOUR GEAR

How you set about organizing your life—and your Zone preparations—over the next four weeks obviously depends on how many decisions you want to make. Some people tell me they just want to follow a detailed plan and not have to make any decisions on their own. Others need to have some flexibility. What's your style? I've got options for you.

Follow My Meal Planner: I recommend this option for busy people who are looking for a no-brainer guaranteed plan. This is true Cruise Control. Simply follow each meal in the Meal Planner as recommended. Use the shopping list to stock up for the week. Some of my most successful clients prepare much of their food ahead of time to make their meals effortless.

Choose Cruise Control–Approved Foods: You'll find extensive food lists starting on page 127. From these approved Cruise Control foods you can create your own meals based on how you are feeling that day. Just remember: limit the Boost Foods to your Boost Zone hours, and then enjoy the Burn beverages and treats in your Burn Zone hours.

Make Cruise Control Recipes: In the next chapter, you'll find more than fifty recipes for meals, snacks, treats, and beverages. You can swap out any meal, snack, or beverage on the food planners with any of these high-octane recipes.

Mix & Match: This choice is all about freedom. If you find you love the exact meal plan of week one but then really like several of my recipes and want to add them to your Boost lineup, go for it! Or you can mix and match from your own Cruise Control–approved creations and the meals and snacks offered. Remember, picking the options you actually love will make this lifestyle enjoyable, which gives you the best chance of success.

AUTOMATE YOUR SCHEDULE

More than twenty years ago, Dr. Oz let me in on a little secret: automation is key to success when incorporating a new lifestyle plan. Take his great advice to heart here. Begin by deciding on the eight-hour Boost Zone and the sixteen-hour Burn Zone windows you think will work best for you. Maybe you're a person who is really in the habit of getting up early and eating something right away. You might not be able to imagine continuing your Burn Zone once you're up and going about your day. If that's the case, you'll want to start your Boost Zone earlier in the day, and also end it earlier—meaning a pretty early dinner and then perhaps having Burn Zone tea or another treat in the early evening hours. Of course, no one has the exact same schedule every day—there will be days that you have a meeting or a social event that requires you to adjust your clock. Life happens! But the more specific and consistent you can be, the better. My husband always says the devil is in the details. That means that trying to anticipate and plan for your daily clock will keep you from getting into the fender benders of life. Remember that sleep is an essential part of your Burn Zone, so those eight hours a night should be penned into your twenty-four-hour schedule as well (you'll find more healthy sleep suggestions on page 254). Get started by filling out the chart below. Don't forget to write in your starting and goal weight.

YOUR CRUISE CONTROL SCHEDULE

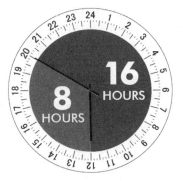

START DATE: _____

GOAL DATE: _____

STARTING WEIGHT: _____
GOAL WEIGHT: _____
TOTAL WEIGHT-LOSS GOAL: _____

YOUR CRUISE CONTROL SCHEDULE

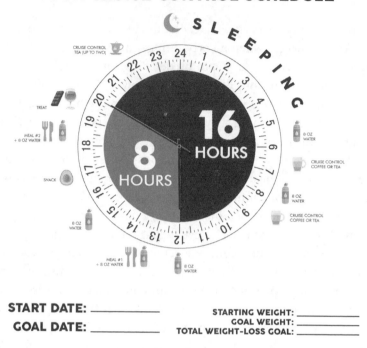

START DATE: _____

GOAL DATE: _____

STARTING WEIGHT: _____
GOAL WEIGHT: _____
TOTAL WEIGHT-LOSS GOAL: _____

But Don't Change Your Life: This might be the most important tip I can offer. Do *not* change your life to fit in Cruise Control. There's no need. You can still live your life without social limitations while being on Cruise Control. There might be times when you can't stay within your eight-hour Boost Zone, or times when you need to break your Burn early—it's no problem. If you are going on a cruise, have holiday parties coming up, or are going to a wedding that will be serving dinner late, relax. You don't need to force a specific Burn or Boost if you have a special occasion to celebrate. Remember, you are in the driver's seat. You can either increase your next Burn Zone or start over with a new eight-hour Boost Zone when you are ready. It's all good.

BURN ZONE RECAP

1. **Drink my Cruise Control Coffee and/or Tea:** There is no limit to the amount of coffee and tea you can drink per day. That said, I recommend that you have all caffeinated beverages before 2:00 P.M., so you don't disrupt your sleep. Dress it up any way you like, with creamer, nondairy or dairy milk, heavy cream, natural sweetener, ghee, grass-fed butter, MCT oil, or coconut oil in your coffee or tea. Only one caveat: no sugar. Staying away from sugar during your Burn Zone keeps your insulin from spiking and helps your body clean up fat storage. You'll find my favorite recipe for Cruise Control Coffee or Tea on page 143.

2. **Drink plenty of water:** Aim to drink a *minimum* of half your body weight in ounces for every twenty-four hours. This will help keep you hydrated and your energy revved, and will keep you feeling full. If you weigh 160 pounds, you'll drink 80 ounces. There are eight ounces in a cup, so you'll drink ten cups of water *minimum* within every twenty-four-hour period. Honor thirst and exercise. If you feel thirsty, drink more. If you sweat a lot due to exercise or heat— drink up again!

3. **Have a set bed and wake time:** Aim for eight to nine hours a night. Remember, you'll be in the Burn Zone during your resting hours. Sleeping and waking at the same time each day will reset your body's clock to accelerate weight loss, improve energy, protect your digestion, help your brain to consolidate memories, and rev up your immune system and your metabolism. You'll be less susceptible to food cravings and overeating, and more likely to feel motivated to stay on Cruise Control. Plus, you'll live longer.

BOOST ZONE RECAP

1. **Eat high-quality fats:** You'll eat 50 percent of your daily nutrients in the form of the best and healthiest fats, oils, and naturally fat-rich whole foods. These include unrefined, organic, and cold-pressed coconut, olive, and avocado oils; organic unsalted and raw nuts and seeds; and organic butter and ghee from grass-fed sources. These

higher-fat foods will get you into the fat-burning zone fast, they'll help you to enhance the absorption of other nutrients during the Boost Zone, and you'll find cravings and hunger extinguished during all twenty-four hours of your day.

2. **Consume lots of vegetables and dark, leafy greens:** These veggies come with the highest amounts of nutrients, antioxidants, and minerals available. They are easy on your digestive system, have hardly any calories, and have lots of fiber.

3. **Keep it low-sugar:** Any refined sugar is something you'll want to minimize. Exceptions are stevia, erythritol, xylitol, or monk fruit. Sugars shut down fat burning and turn on fat storage. It's effortless. Simply follow my food planner in the next chapter.

4. **Drink water:** Just as with the Burn Zone, you'll drink plenty of water. I recommend adding lemons or limes to your water to balance your gut's microbiome.

5. **Focus on eating real, unprocessed foods:** The Cruise Control meal plan is devoid of all refined and processed foods and sugars.

6. **Enjoy your favorite carbs!** Bread, pasta, and rice are permitted in moderation. Carbohydrates are broken down into sugar, so the more you avoid these foods, the better your results. Note: whole-grain and organic are best.

7. **Include wine and desserts if you really want to:** On the Cruise Control plan you are allowed to indulge in wine (organic, sulfite-free is best) up to three times per week, and plan on enjoying dessert daily. Let me tell you about a dessert hack I love. I am hooked on ice creams by Killer Creamery. They make the most delicious, creamy concoctions that are made from cream and pure coconut MCT oil. Plus, they have no sugar added. They use only Cruise Control–approved sweeteners erythritol and stevia. You can find out more about these guys, where to buy them, and flavors available on page 305. Choose from their low carb/keto flavors of ice cream.

8. **Use organic Himalayan pink salt:** Add a pinch of organic Himalayan pink salt or other high-mineral salts to your coffee, water, and food. Salt is full of minerals that promote cellular hydration.

SHOP, PREP, EAT!

So, you're all geared up and have made some decisions—as best you can—about how you want to organize your Burn and Boost Zones for the next four weeks. If you're going to let me take the lead and you plan to follow my exact regimen, take a look below at exactly what you'll need to buy and have on hand to eat in the coming weeks and the combinations in which you'll cook and devour all this good nutrition!

Meal Planner: Week One

WEEK ONE SHOPPING LIST

PRODUCE

Arugula—5 cups
Avocado—¾ cup
Bell pepper—5
Cilantro
Cucumber
Garlic
Ginger
Kale—3 cups
Lemon—3
Lettuce—3 cups
Mushroom—9
Red onion
Rosemary
Red cabbage—1
Spinach
Tomato—3
White onion—1

PROTEIN

Egg—2 large
Grilled chicken—15 ounces

Steak—Two 3-ounce pieces
Shrimp—6 ounces

DAIRY

Grated mozzarella cheese—3 ounces
Greek yogurt—2 ounces
Parmesan cheese—3 ounces
Whipped cream—6 tablespoons

OTHER

Apple cider vinegar
Almonds—36
Almond butter—6 tablespoons
Balsamic vinegar
Black pepper
Cauliflower rice—2 cups
Cayenne pepper
Extra-virgin olive oil
Ground espresso
Olives—4 ounces
Paprika
Peanuts—2 teaspoons
Salt
Turmeric
Walnuts—4
Whole-wheat tortillas—2
Three 4-ounce glasses of red wine *OR* 9 squares of 85% pure dark
    cocoa bar
3 squares of 85% pure dark cocoa bar
Cruise Control Coffee and/or Tea

DAY ONE

ZONE	FOOD	NOTES
Burn: Morning	Cruise Control Coffee (or Tea)	Enjoy up to 3 servings before lunch.
Boost: Lunch	Lemon Chicken Kale Salad	1 cup lettuce and 1 cup kale tossed with 3 ounces grilled chicken, ⅛ cup Parmesan cheese, fresh pepper, and juice and zest from 1 lemon.
Boost: Snack	Kalamata Olives	⅛ cup kalamata olives.
Boost: Dinner	Zesty Portobello Pizza	Remove gills and stem of 1 portobello mushroom and season with salt, pepper, and cayenne, then bake at 400°F for 5 minutes. Blend 1 tomato with ½ bell pepper, 1 clove garlic, and 1 teaspoon olive oil until smooth. Top mushroom with sauce and ⅛ cup grated mozzarella cheese. Return to oven and bake until the cheese is melted. Serve with 1 cup arugula tossed in balsamic vinegar.
Boost: Treat	Wine or Chocolate	One 4-ounce glass red wine *or* 1 serving (3 squares) 85% pure dark cocoa.

DAY TWO

ZONE	FOOD	NOTES
Burn: Morning	Cruise Control Coffee (or Tea)	Enjoy up to 3 servings before lunch.
Boost: Lunch	Warm Spinach Salad	Quickly sauté 2 cups spinach with balsamic vinegar and sliced red onion. Serve with 2 chopped walnuts, 3 sliced mushrooms, and 1 egg over easy. Sprinkle with balsamic vinegar and fresh pepper.
Boost: Snack	Peppers and Avocado	1 cup sliced bell peppers and ¼ cup mashed avocado seasoned with lemon juice, salt, and pepper.
Boost: Dinner	Espresso Rubbed Steak and Rosemary Cauliflower Rice	Rub 3 ounces steak with ground espresso, garlic, and pepper, then grill. Serve with 1 cup cauliflower rice seasoned with rosemary and cayenne pepper. Toss 1 cup arugula with lemon juice.
Boost: Treat	Almond Butter and Almonds	2 tablespoons almond butter topped with 2 tablespoons whipped cream and 6 almonds.

DAY THREE

ZONE	FOOD	NOTES
Burn: Morning	Cruise Control Coffee (or Tea)	Enjoy up to 3 servings before lunch.
Boost: Lunch	Lemon Chicken Kale Salad	1 cup lettuce and 1 cup kale tossed with 3 ounces grilled chicken, ⅛ cup Parmesan cheese, fresh pepper, and juice and zest from 1 lemon.
Boost: Snack	Kalamata Olives	⅛ cup kalamata olives.
Boost: Dinner	Turmeric Shrimp Fajitas	Grill 3 ounces shrimp seasoned with turmeric and paprika. Assemble fajitas in a whole-wheat tortilla topped with shrimp, sautéed bell pepper, onions, and chopped spinach. Drizzle top with ⅛ cup Greek yogurt mixed with chopped cilantro.
Boost: Treat	Wine or Chocolate	One 4-ounce glass red wine *or* 1 serving (3 squares) 85% pure dark cocoa.

DAY FOUR

ZONE	FOOD	NOTES
Burn: Morning	Cruise Control Coffee (or Tea)	Enjoy up to 3 servings before lunch.
Boost: Lunch	Ginger Chicken Cabbage Slaw	Season 3 ounces chicken with lemon and ginger, and grill. Shred ½ small red cabbage, and finely slice onion and cucumber. Toss with apple cider vinegar, and garnish with 1 teaspoon each of chopped peanuts and cilantro.
Boost: Snack	Peppers and Avocado	1 cup sliced bell peppers with ¼ cup mashed avocado seasoned with lemon juice, salt, and pepper.
Boost: Dinner	Zesty Portobello Pizza	Remove gills and stem of 1 portobello mushroom and season with salt, pepper, and cayenne, then bake at 400°F for 5 minutes. Blend 1 tomato with ½ bell pepper, 1 clove garlic, and 1 teaspoon olive oil until smooth. Top mushroom with sauce and ⅛ cup grated mozzarella cheese. Return to oven and bake until the cheese melts. Serve with 1 cup arugula tossed in balsamic vinegar.
Boost: Treat	Almond Butter and Almonds	2 tablespoons almond butter topped with 2 tablespoons whipped cream and 6 almonds.

DAY FIVE

ZONE	FOOD	NOTES
Burn: Morning	Cruise Control Coffee (or Tea)	Enjoy up to 3 servings before lunch.
Boost: Lunch	Lemon Chicken Kale Salad	1 cup lettuce and 1 cup kale tossed with 3 ounces grilled chicken, ⅛ cup Parmesan cheese, fresh pepper, and juice and zest from 1 lemon.
Boost: Snack	Kalamata Olives	⅛ cup kalamata olives.
Boost: Dinner	Espresso Rubbed Steak and Rosemary Cauliflower Rice	Rub 3 ounces steak with ground espresso, garlic, and pepper, then grill. Serve with 1 cup cauliflower rice seasoned with rosemary and cayenne pepper. Toss 1 cup arugula with lemon juice.
Boost: Treat	Wine or Chocolate	One 4-ounce glass red wine or 1 serving (3 squares) 85% pure dark cocoa.

DAY SIX

ZONE	FOOD	NOTES
Burn: Morning	Cruise Control Coffee (or Tea)	Enjoy up to 3 servings before lunch.
Boost: Lunch	Warm Spinach Salad	Quickly sauté 2 cups spinach with balsamic vinegar and sliced red onion. Serve with 2 chopped walnuts, 3 sliced mushrooms, and 1 egg over easy. Sprinkle balsamic vinegar and fresh pepper on top.
Boost: Snack	Peppers and Avocado	1 cup sliced bell peppers with ¼ cup mashed avocado seasoned with lemon juice, salt, and pepper.
Boost: Dinner	Turmeric Shrimp Fajitas	Grill 3 ounces shrimp seasoned with turmeric and paprika. Assemble fajitas in a whole-wheat tortilla topped with shrimp, sautéed bell pepper, onions, and spinach. Drizzle top with ⅛ cup Greek yogurt mixed with chopped cilantro.
Boost: Treat	Almond Butter or Almonds	2 tablespoons almond butter topped with 2 tablespoons whipped cream and 6 almonds.

DAY SEVEN

ZONE	FOOD	NOTES
Burn: Morning	Cruise Control Coffee (or Tea)	Enjoy up to 3 servings before lunch.
Boost: Lunch	Ginger Chicken Cabbage Slaw	Season 3 ounces chicken with lemon and ginger and grill. Shred ½ small red cabbage, finely sliced onion, and cucumber. Toss with apple cider vinegar and garnish with 1 teaspoon chopped peanuts and cilantro.
Boost: Snack	Kalamata Olives	⅛ cup kalamata olives.
Boost: Dinner	Zesty Portobello Pizza	Remove gills and stem of 1 portobello mushroom and season with salt, pepper, and cayenne, then bake at 400°F for 5 minutes. Blend 1 tomato with ½ bell pepper, 1 clove garlic, and 1 teaspoon olive oil until smooth. Top mushroom with sauce and ⅛ cup grated mozzarella cheese. Return to oven and bake until the cheese melts. Serve with 1 cup of arugula tossed in balsamic vinegar.
Boost: Treat	Chocolate	1 serving (3 squares) 85% pure dark cocoa.

WEEK TWO SHOPPING LIST

PRODUCE

Avocados—2
Asparagus—9 spears
Basil
Bell pepper—¾ cup
Garlic
Grapes—1 cup
Lime
Mushrooms—1 cup
Parsley
Romaine lettuce
Spinach—2 cups
Tomatoes—4

PROTEIN

Bacon—3 slices
Deli turkey—3 slices
Eggs—6 large
Shrimp—6 ounces
Skinny steak—Two 3-ounce pieces

DAIRY

Blue cheese—2 tablespoons
Parmesan cheese—5 teaspoons
Swiss cheese—3 slices
String cheese—3 ounces
Mozzarella cheese—8 ounces
Unsalted butter—2 tablespoons

OTHER

Balsamic vinegar
Black beans—1½ cups
Chili pepper
Corn tortillas—2
Granulated natural sugar (erythritol)—6 tablespoons
Ground pepper
Peanut butter (creamy, low-sugar)—6 tablespoons
Ranch dressing
Salt
Zucchini noodles—6 cups
Six 4-ounce glasses of Pinot Noir *or* 3 cups frozen grapes
Cruise Control Coffee and/or Tea

DAY ONE

ZONE	FOOD	NOTES
Burn: Morning	Cruise Control Coffee (or Tea)	Enjoy up to 3 servings before lunch.
Boost: Lunch	Turkey Lettuce Wrap	In a romaine lettuce leaf, layer 1 slice deli turkey, 1 slice Swiss cheese, ¼ cup diced tomatoes, ¼ cup sliced bell pepper, and 1 teaspoon ranch dressing.
Boost: Snack	Avocado	½ cup cubed avocado topped with cracked pepper and a pinch of salt.
Boost: Dinner	Bacon-Wrapped Asparagus with Egg	Wrap 3 spears of asparagus with a slice of bacon and bake at 400°F for 15 to 20 minutes or until desired crispness. Top bacon-wrapped asparagus with 1 egg (poached, soft-boiled, or over easy) and 1 teaspoon Parmesan cheese.
Boost: Treat	Wine or Frozen Grapes	Two 4-ounce glasses Pinot Noir or 1 cup frozen grapes.

DAY TWO

ZONE	FOOD	NOTES
Burn: Morning	Cruise Control Coffee (or Tea)	Enjoy up to 3 servings before lunch.
Boost: Lunch	Bruschetta Stack	Slice 1 tomato and 4 ounces mozzarella cheese into thick slices. Layer 1 tomato slice, cheese, then top with basil leaves and a drizzle of balsamic vinegar. Sprinkle with pepper.
Boost: Snack	String Cheese	1 ounce string cheese.
Boost: Dinner	Garlic Shrimp Pasta	Sauté 3 ounces shrimp in 1 tablespoon unsalted butter and 2 minced cloves of garlic. Add to 3 cups zucchini noodles and top with chopped parsley and 1 teaspoon Parmesan cheese.
Boost: Treat	Cruise PB Cake	Whisk 2 tablespoons low-sugar creamy peanut butter, 2 teaspoons granulated natural sweetener (erythritol), and 1 large egg into a microwave-safe mug until it reaches a creamy consistency. Microwave for 1 minute. Let it cool down before eating. Top with 2 tablespoons whipped cream.

DAY THREE

ZONE	FOOD	NOTES
Burn: Morning	Cruise Control Coffee (or Tea)	Enjoy up to 3 servings before lunch.
Boost: Lunch	Turkey Lettuce Wrap	In a romaine lettuce leaf, layer 1 slice deli turkey, 1 slice Swiss cheese, ¼ cup diced tomatoes, ¼ cup sliced bell pepper, and 1 teaspoon ranch dressing.
Boost: Snack	Avocado	½ cup cubed avocado topped with cracked pepper and a pinch of salt.
Boost: Dinner	Blue Cheese Mushroom Steak	Grill 3 ounces skirt steak seasoned with chili pepper, salt, and pepper. Serve with 1 cup wilted spinach, ½ cup sautéed mushrooms, and 1 tablespoon blue cheese.
Boost: Treat	Wine or Frozen Grapes	Two 4-ounce glasses Pinot Noir *or* 1 cup frozen grapes.

DAY FOUR

ZONE	FOOD	NOTES
Burn: Morning	Cruise Control Coffee (or Tea)	Enjoy up to 3 servings before lunch.
Boost: Lunch	Fresh Fiesta Tacos	Mix ¾ cup black beans with ½ cup diced tomatoes, salt, pepper, and lime juice. Fill warm corn tortilla with mixture, and top with chopped cilantro.
Boost: Snack	String Cheese	1 ounce string cheese.
Boost: Dinner	Bacon-Wrapped Asparagus with Egg	Wrap 3 spears asparagus with 1 slice of bacon, and bake at 400°F for 15 to 20 minutes or until desired crispness. Top bacon-wrapped asparagus with 1 egg (poached, soft-boiled, or over easy) and 1 teaspoon Parmesan cheese.
Boost: Treat	Cruise PB Cake	Whisk 2 tablespoons low-sugar creamy peanut butter, 2 tablespoons granulated natural sweetener (erythritol), and 1 large egg into a microwave-safe mug until it reaches a creamy consistency. Microwave for 1 minute. Let it cool down before eating. Top with 2 tablespoons whipped cream.

DAY FIVE

ZONE	FOOD	NOTES
Burn: Morning	Cruise Control Coffee (or Tea)	Enjoy up to 3 servings before lunch.
Boost: Lunch	Turkey Lettuce Wrap	In a romaine lettuce leaf, layer 1 slice deli turkey, 1 slice Swiss cheese, ¼ cup diced tomatoes, ¼ cup sliced bell pepper, and 1 teaspoon ranch dressing.
Boost: Snack	Avocado	½ cup cubed avocado topped with cracked pepper and a pinch of salt.
Boost: Dinner	Garlic Shrimp Pasta	Sauté 3 ounces shrimp in 1 tablespoon unsalted butter and 2 minced cloves of garlic. Add to 3 cups zucchini noodles and top with chopped parsley and 1 teaspoon Parmesan cheese.
Boost: Treat	Wine or Frozen Grapes	Two 4-ounce glasses Pinot Noir or 1 cup frozen grapes.

DAY SIX

ZONE	FOOD	NOTES
Burn: Morning	Cruise Control Coffee (or Tea)	Enjoy up to 3 servings before lunch.
Boost: Lunch	Bruschetta Stack	Slice 1 tomato and 4 ounces mozzarella cheese into thick slices. Layer tomato slice, cheese, and top with basil leaves and a drizzle of balsamic vinegar. Sprinkle with pepper.
Boost: Snack	String Cheese	1 ounce string cheese.
Boost: Dinner	Blue Cheese Mushroom Steak	Grill 3 ounces skirt steak seasoned with chili pepper, salt, and pepper. Serve with 1 cup wilted spinach, ½ cup sautéed mushrooms, and 1 tablespoon blue cheese.
Boost: Treat	Cruise PB Cake	Whisk 2 tablespoons low-sugar creamy peanut butter, 2 tablespoons granulated natural sweetener (erythritol), and 1 large egg into a microwave-safe mug until it reaches a creamy consistency. Microwave for 1 minute. Let it cool down before eating. Top with 2 tablespoons whipped cream.

DAY SEVEN

ZONE	FOOD	NOTES
Burn: Morning	Cruise Control Coffee (or Tea)	Enjoy up to 3 servings before lunch.
Boost: Lunch	Fresh Fiesta Tacos	Mix ¾ cup black beans with ½ cup diced tomatoes, salt, pepper, and lime juice. Fill warm corn tortilla with mixture and top with chopped cilantro.
Boost: Snack	Avocado	½ cup of cubed avocado topped with cracked pepper and a pinch of salt.
Boost: Dinner	Bacon-Wrapped Asparagus with Egg	Wrap 3 spears asparagus with 1 slice of bacon, and bake at 400°F for 15 to 20 minutes or until desired crispness. Top bacon-wrapped asparagus with 1 egg (poached, soft boiled, or over easy) and 1 teaspoon Parmesan cheese.
Boost: Treat	Frozen Grapes	1 cup frozen grapes.

WEEK THREE SHOPPING LIST

PRODUCE

Arugula—4 cups
Avocado—1 cup
Bell pepper
Butternut squash—3 cups
Carrot—1
Cilantro
Cremini mushroom—1
Cucumber—3 slices
Ginger—1 teaspoon
Green onion—2
Lettuce leaves—4
Onion
Red chili—2
Romaine lettuce—6 cups
Spinach—2 cup
Strawberries—5 cups
Swiss chard—6 cups

PROTEIN

Chicken—Seven 3-ounce pieces
Ground turkey—6 ounces
Steak—Three 3-ounce pieces

DAIRY

Feta cheese—3 ounces
Grated mozzarella cheese—2 ounces
Parmesan cheese—2 ounces
Whipped cream

OTHER

Almonds—18 raw, dry-roasted, smoked
Balsamic vinegar
Chicken stock—2 cups
Chili powder
Coconut milk—4 teaspoons
Coriander
Cumin
Lemon juice
Macadamia nuts—3 tablespoons
Pecans—2 tablespoons
Pepper
Pork rinds—4 cups
Thyme
Tomato sauce—1 cup
Zucchini noodles—1 cup
9 squares 85% pure dark cocoa bar
Cruise Control Coffee and/or Tea

DAY ONE

ZONE	FOOD	NOTES
Burn: Morning	Cruise Control Coffee (or Tea)	Enjoy up to 3 servings before lunch.
Boost: Lunch	Greek Chicken Salad	2 cups romaine lettuce, 3 ounces chicken, 1 ounce feta cheese, and 1 sliced cucumber tossed with lemon juice.
Boost: Snack	Pork Rinds	1 cup pork rinds.
Boost: Dinner	Butternut Squash with Steak	1 cup sautéed butternut squash with 2 cups Swiss chard, seasoned with thyme. Serve with 3 ounces steak seasoned with pepper and cumin.
Boost: Treat	Strawberries and Whipped Cream	1 cup strawberries with 1 table-spoon whipped cream.

DAY TWO

ZONE	FOOD	NOTES
Burn: Morning	Cruise Control Coffee (or Tea)	Enjoy up to 3 servings before lunch.
Boost: Lunch	Thai Chicken Soup	Sauté 3 ounces cubed chicken in a saucepan, then add 1 cup chicken stock, 1 small diced red chili, and ½ teaspoon grated ginger. Bring to a boil, then add 2 tablespoons coconut milk, 1 sliced green onion, ½ cup sliced cremini mushrooms, and chopped cilantro.
Boost: Snack	Macadamia Nuts	1 tablespoon macadamia nuts.
Boost: Dinner	Chicken Zoodles	Zucchini noodles with ½ cup tomato sauce, and 3 ounces chicken topped with 1 ounce Parmesan cheese. Serve with 1 cup spinach tossed in balsamic vinegar.
Boost: Treat	Chocolate and Almonds	1 serving (3 squares) 85% pure dark cocoa with 6 almonds.

DAY THREE

ZONE	FOOD	NOTES
Burn: Morning	Cruise Control Coffee (or Tea)	Enjoy up to 3 servings before lunch.
Boost: Lunch	Greek Chicken Salad	2 cups romaine lettuce, 3 ounces chicken, 1 ounce feta cheese, and 1 sliced cucumber tossed with lemon juice.
Boost: Snack	Pork Rinds	1 cup pork rinds.
Boost: Dinner	Turkey Lettuce Tacos	3 ounces ground turkey seasoned with coriander and chili powder. Fill 2 leaves of lettuce with meat, 1 ounce grated mozzarella cheese, diced onion, 1 grated carrot, and bell pepper.
Boost: Treat	Strawberries and Whipped Cream	1 cup strawberries with 1 tablespoon whipped cream.

DAY FOUR

ZONE	FOOD	NOTES
Burn: Morning	Cruise Control Coffee (or Tea)	Enjoy up to 3 servings before lunch.
Boost: Lunch	Spring Berry Salad	2 cups arugula tossed with ½ cup sliced strawberries, ½ cup diced avocado, and 1 tablespoon chopped pecans drizzled with balsamic vinegar.
Boost: Snack	Macadamia Nuts	1 tablespoon macadamia nuts.
Boost: Dinner	Butternut Squash with Steak	1 cup sautéed butternut squash with 2 cups Swiss chard seasoned with thyme. Serve with 3 ounces steak seasoned with pepper and cumin.
Boost: Treat	Chocolate and Almonds	1 serving (3 squares) 85% pure dark cocoa with 6 almonds.

DAY FIVE

ZONE	FOOD	NOTES
Burn: Morning	Cruise Control Coffee (or Tea)	Enjoy up to 3 servings before lunch.
Boost: Lunch	Greek Chicken Salad	2 cups romaine lettuce, 3 ounces chicken, 1 ounce feta cheese, and 1 sliced cucumber tossed with lemon juice.
Boost: Snack	Pork Rinds	1 cup pork rinds.
Boost: Dinner	Chicken Zoodles	Zucchini noodles with ½ cup tomato sauce, and 3 ounces chicken topped with 1 ounce Parmesan cheese. Serve with 1 cup spinach tossed in balsamic vinegar.
Boost: Treat	Strawberries and Whipped Cream	1 cup strawberries with 1 tablespoon whipped cream.

DAY SIX

ZONE	FOOD	NOTES
Burn: Morning	Cruise Control Coffee (or Tea)	Enjoy up to 3 servings before lunch.
Boost: Lunch	Thai Chicken Soup	Sauté 3 ounces cubed chicken in a saucepan, then add 1 cup chicken stock, 1 small diced red chili, and ½ teaspoon grated ginger. Bring to a boil, then add 2 tablespoons coconut milk, 1 sliced green onion, ½ cup sliced cremini mushrooms, and chopped cilantro.
Boost: Snack	Macadamia Nuts	1 tablespoon macadamia nuts.
Boost: Dinner	Turkey Lettuce Tacos	3 ounces ground turkey seasoned with coriander and chili powder. Fill 2 leaves of lettuce with meat, 1 ounce grated mozzarella cheese, diced onion, 1 grated carrot, and bell pepper.
Boost: Treat	Chocolate and Almonds	1 serving (3 squares) 85% pure dark cocoa with 6 almonds.

DAY SEVEN

ZONE	FOOD	NOTES
Burn: Morning	Cruise Control Coffee (or Tea)	Enjoy up to 3 servings before lunch.
Boost: Lunch	Spring Berry Salad	2 cups arugula tossed with ½ cup sliced strawberries, ½ cup diced avocado, and 1 tablespoon chopped pecans drizzled with balsamic vinegar.
Boost: Snack	Pork Rinds	1 cup pork rinds.
Boost: Dinner	Butternut Squash with Steak	1 cup sautéed butternut squash with 2 cups Swiss chard, seasoned with thyme. Serve with 3 ounces steak seasoned with pepper and cumin.
Boost: Treat	Strawberries and Whipped Cream	1 cup strawberries with 1 tablespoon whipped cream.

WEEK FOUR SHOPPING LIST

PRODUCE

Arugula—6 cups
Avocados—1½
Beets—7
Carrot
Celery
Cucumber
Dates—3
Eggplant—2
Endive
Garlic
Ginger
Green onion
Kale—4 cups
Lemon
Lettuce—1 head
Parsley
Roasted chickpeas—8 ounces
Tomatoes—3
Zucchini

PROTEIN

Almonds (dry roasted or smoked, but not candied)
Bacon—9 strips
Chicken—Three 3-ounce pieces
Eggs—3 large
Ground beef—3 patties
Ground turkey—9 ounces
Parmesan cheese—3 ounces

DAIRY

Cheddar cheese—½ cup
Swiss cheese—6 slices

OTHER

Balsamic vinegar
Barbecue sauce—2 teaspoons
Brown rice—⅔ cup
Cumin
Merlot—Six 4-ounce cups *or* 9 dates
Mustard
Orange juice—1 cup
Paprika
Pepper
Pesto
Quinoa—1 cup
Salt
Sesame seeds
Soy sauce—2 teaspoons
Whole-wheat or gluten-free bread—2 slices
Worcestershire sauce
Cruise Control Coffee and/or Tea

DAY ONE

ZONE	FOOD	NOTES
Burn: Morning	Cruise Control Coffee (or Tea)	Enjoy up to 3 servings before lunch.
Boost: Lunch	Cruise Cheeseburger	1 hamburger spread with 1 teaspoon mustard, 2 slices Swiss cheese, ½ avocado smashed, and 3 strips bacon in lettuce.
Boost: Snack	Chickpeas	2 ounces roasted chickpeas seasoned with paprika.
Boost: Dinner	Parmesan-Crusted Chicken with Arugula	Dip 3 ounces chicken in 1 beaten egg, and then coat in 1 ounce Parmesan cheese mixed with parsley, lemon zest, and garlic. In a hot skillet, brown both sides, then reduce heat to low and cover. Cook for about 10 minutes with the lid on. Serve with 2 cups arugula tossed in mustard, balsamic vinegar, and 1 diced tomato.
Boost: Treat	Wine or Dates	Two 4-ounce glasses Merlot or 3 dates.

DAY TWO

ZONE	FOOD	NOTES
Burn: Morning	Cruise Control Coffee (or Tea)	Enjoy up to 3 servings before lunch.
Boost: Lunch	Ginger Quinoa Kale Salad	2 cups kale tossed with grated beet, grated carrot, 1 diced celery, and ½ cup quinoa. Add grated ginger and lemon juice.
Boost: Snack	Roasted Beet Chips	Thinly slice 2 beets, season with salt, pepper, and cumin, and roast until crisp.
Boost: Dinner	Zucchini Boats	Halve a large zucchini and scoop out the seeds. Mix 3 ounces cooked ground turkey with 1 tablespoon barbecue sauce, salt, and pepper, then place on zucchini boats. Top with ¼ cup grated Cheddar cheese and bake at 400°F until the cheese is melted.
Boost: Treat	Smoked Almonds	5 raw, dry-roasted, smoked almonds.

DAY THREE

ZONE	FOOD	NOTES
Burn: Morning	Cruise Control Coffee (or Tea)	Enjoy up to 3 servings before lunch.
Boost: Lunch	Cruise Cheese-burger	1 hamburger spread with 1 teaspoon mustard, 2 slices Swiss cheese, ½ avocado smashed, and 3 strips bacon in lettuce.
Boost: Snack	Chickpeas	2 ounces roasted chickpeas seasoned with paprika.
Boost: Dinner	Orange Eggplant with Brown Rice	Cube 1 eggplant and marinate in ½ cup orange juice, ginger, garlic, 1 teaspoon soy sauce, and Worcestershire. Sauté over high heat until crispy and cooked through. Add sliced green onions, 1 teaspoon sesame seeds, and sliced endive. Serve on top of ⅓ cup brown rice.
Boost: Treat	Wine or Dates	Two 4-ounce glasses Merlot *or* 3 dates.

DAY FOUR

ZONE	FOOD	NOTES
Burn: Morning	Cruise Control Coffee (or Tea)	Enjoy up to 3 servings before lunch.
Boost: Lunch	Turkey Cucumber Sandwich	Toast 1 slice whole-wheat or gluten-free bread, then layer 3 ounces turkey, sliced cucumber, kale, and pesto. Serve with 1 cup lettuce tossed in lemon juice and pepper.
Boost: Snack	Roasted Beet Chips	Thinly slice 2 beets, season with salt, pepper, and cumin, and roast until crisp.
Boost: Dinner	Parmesan-Crusted Chicken with Arugula	Dip 3 ounces chicken in 1 beaten egg and then coat in 1 ounce Parmesan cheese mixed with parsley, lemon zest, and garlic. In a hot skillet, brown both sides, then reduce heat to low and cover. Let cook for about 10 minutes with the lid on. Serve with 2 cups arugula tossed in mustard, balsamic vinegar, and 1 diced tomato.
Boost: Treat	Smoked Almonds	15 dry roasted or smoked almonds.

DAY FIVE

ZONE	FOOD	NOTES
Burn: Morning	Cruise Control Coffee (or Tea)	Enjoy up to 3 servings before lunch.
Boost: Lunch	Cruise Cheeseburger	One hamburger spread with 1 teaspoon mustard, 2 slices Swiss cheese, ½ avocado smashed, and 3 strips of bacon in lettuce.
Boost: Snack	Roasted Chickpeas	2 ounces roasted chickpeas seasoned with paprika.
Boost: Dinner	Zucchini Boats	Halve a large zucchini and scoop out the seeds. Mix 3 ounces cooked ground turkey with 1 tablespoon barbecue sauce, salt, and pepper, then place on zucchini boats. Top with ¼ cup grated Cheddar cheese and bake at 400°F until the cheese melts.
Boost: Treat	Wine or Dates	Two 4-ounce glasses Merlot *or* 3 dates.

DAY SIX

ZONE	FOOD	NOTES
Burn: Morning	Cruise Control Coffee (or Tea)	Enjoy up to 3 servings before lunch.
Boost: Lunch	Ginger Quinoa Kale Salad	2 cups of kale tossed with grated beet, grated carrot, 1 diced celery, and ½ cup quinoa. Add grated ginger and lemon juice.
Boost: Snack	Roasted Beet Chips	Thinly slice 2 beets, season with salt, pepper, and cumin, and roast until crisp.
Boost: Dinner	Orange Eggplant with Brown Rice	Cube 1 eggplant and marinate in ½ cup orange juice, ginger, garlic, 1 teaspoon soy sauce, and Worcestershire. Sauté over high heat until crispy and cooked through. Add sliced green onions, 1 teaspoon sesame seeds, and sliced endive. Serve on top of ⅓ cup brown rice.
Boost: Treat	Smoked Almonds	15 dry roasted or smoked almonds.

DAY SEVEN

ZONE	FOOD	NOTES
Burn: Morning	Cruise Control Coffee (or Tea)	Enjoy up to 3 servings before lunch.
Boost: Lunch	Turkey Cucumber Sandwich	Toast 1 slice whole-wheat or gluten-free bread, then layer 3 ounces turkey, sliced cucumber, kale, and pesto. Serve with 1 cup lettuce tossed in lemon juice and pepper.
Boost: Snack	Roasted Chickpeas	2 ounces roasted chickpeas seasoned with paprika.
Boost: Dinner	Parmesan-Crusted Chicken with Arugula	Dip 3 ounces chicken in 1 beaten egg and then coat in 1 ounce shredded Parmesan cheese mixed with parsley, lemon zest, and garlic. In a hot skillet, brown both sides, then reduce heat to low and cover. Let cook for about 10 minutes with the lid on. Serve with 2 cups arugula tossed in mustard, balsamic vinegar, and 1 diced tomato.
Boost: Treat	Dates	3 dates.

A Note about Substitutions

I know you are busy, so I designed these four-week meal planners to be quick toss-together meals. After all, I want healthy eating to be an entirely uncomplicated and pressure-free activity for you. At the same time, there is nothing like a more involved homemade meal to make you feel genuinely nourished and together. In the next chapter, you'll find more than fifty recipes that you can use as substitutes for any item on the four-week meal planners above (as long as it fits the Boost Zone or Burn Zone, respectively).

Approved Foods List

If you've decided that you want to create your own meals (or mix and match from your own repertoire and from my meal plans above), you're going to need to know exactly what to put in your shopping cart. Toward that end, I have created the following food lists to help you on the path to success in both your Burn and Boost Zones. The only rule with the Burn Zone beverages and treats is to enjoy them whenever you feel like it. They can be consumed whether you are within your eight-hour Boost Zone or the sixteen-hour Burn Zone. How great is that?

The Boost Zone meals and snacks need to be consumed within your eight-hour window each day. All of these foods will help supercharge your weight loss because they keep insulin at low levels, which means you can burn fat at higher rates for more hours each day. These are the foods that will make up the foundation of your daily eating plan, and you'll see all these foods incorporated into the meal planners. This strategy also keeps you from having uncontrollable cravings that can sabotage your efforts. Remember, when insulin is spiked, as it is with highly refined, easily digestible sugars and starches, it causes your body to store its fuel as fat, it makes you hungrier faster than low-insulin foods will, and it causes cravings for more of the same unhealthy foods. These foods will keep you Cruising.

Look for * next to foods that are Burn-Zone-safe; check meal planners for serving sizes.

BEVERAGES

Bone broth*
Coffee*
Carbonated water*
Heavy cream*
Purified water*
Sparkling water*
Stevia-sweetened sugar-free sodas*
Tea (herbal, unsweetened, green, oolong, eleotin, and yerba mate)*
Unsweetened almond milk*
Unsweetened coconut milk*
Unsweetened half-and-half*
Unsweetened nut milk*
Water*

OILS & FATS

Almond oil*
Avocado oil*
Avocado oil mayo
Balsamic vinegar
Butter*
Cacao butter/oil*
Chia seed oil*
Coconut cream*
Coconut oil*
Dark chocolate
Extra-virgin olive oil*
Fish oil*
Flaxseed oil*
Flaxseeds
Grass-fed butter*
Grass-fed ghee*
Hazelnut oil*

Heavy cream*
Hemp seed oil*
Krill oil*
Macadamia nut oil*
MCT oil*
Palm fruit oil*
Palm kernel oil*
Sesame oil*
Spirulina
Walnut oil*

SPICES & FLAVORINGS

Apple cider vinegar
Balsamic vinegar
Basil
Black pepper
Cayenne pepper*
Chamomile*
Chili powder
Chives
Cilantro
Cinnamon*
Cumin
Curry powder
Dill
Garlic
Ginger*
Himalayan pink salt*
Horseradish
Hot sauce
Lemon*
Lime*
Mayonnaise
Mint*
Mustard*
Nutmeg ground*
Oregano

Parsley
Pepper*
Peppermint*
Red pepper flakes
Rosemary
Sage
Sea salt*
Thyme
Turmeric*

SWEETENERS

Erythritol*
Monk fruit*
Stevia*
Swerve*
Xylitol*

ORGANIC VEGETABLES

Artichoke
Arugula
Asparagus
Beets
Bell peppers
Bok choy
Broccoli
Brussels sprouts
Butternut squash
Cabbage
Carrots
Cauliflower
Celery
Chickpeas
Collard greens
Cucumbers
Dill pickles

Eggplant
Endive
Fennel
Garlic
Green beans
Kale
Lettuce
Mushrooms
Olives
Onions
Peas
Peppers
Pickles
Pumpkin
Radicchio
Radishes
Sauerkraut
Scallions
Seaweed
Shallots
Snap peas
Spinach
Squash
Tomato
Zucchini

NUTS, SEEDS, & LEGUMES

Almond butter
Almonds
Brazil nuts
Cashews
Chia seeds
Coconut
Coconut butter
Flaxseeds
Hazelnuts
Hemp seeds

Macadamia nuts
Pecans
Pine nuts
Pistachios
Pumpkin seeds
Sesame seeds
Sunflower seeds
Walnuts

DAIRY

American cheese
Asiago cheese
Blue cheese
Brick cheese
Brie cheese
Cheddar cheese
Chèvre cheese
Colby cheese
Colby Jack cheese
Colostrum
Cottage cheese (organic full-fat)
Cream
Feta cheese
Fontina cheese
Full-fat yogurt
Goat cheese
Gorgonzola cheese
Gouda cheese
Grass-fed butter
Greek yogurt
Havarti cheese
Heavy cream*
Jack cheese
Manchego cheese
Monterey Jack cheese
Mozzarella cheese
Parmesan cheese

Pepper Jack cheese
Provolone cheese
Ricotta cheese
Romano cheese
Sour cream
Swiss cheese
Unsweetened almond milk*
Unsweetened coconut milk*
Unsweetened half-and-half*
Unsweetened nut milk*
Whipped cream*

PROTEIN

Anchovies
Bacon
Bass
Beef jerky
Bologna
Bone broth protein
Buffalo
Catfish
Chicken
Chorizo
Clams
Cod
Collagen protein
Crab
Duck
Egg protein
Eggs, large
Flounder
Goose
Grass-fed beef
Grass-fed lamb
Grass-fed steak
Grass-fed whey protein
Ground beef

Halibut
Ham
Lamb
Lobster
Mahimahi
Ocean perch
Oysters
Pastured eggs cage-free, large
Pastured duck
Pastured goose
Pastured pork
Pepperoni
Pork
Prosciutto
Salami
Salmon
Sardines
Sausage
Scallops
Shrimp
Snapper
Sole
Swordfish
Tilapia
Tofu
Trout
Turkey
Tuna
Veal

STARCH

Acorn squash
Barley
Black rice
Brown rice
Buckwheat
Butternut squash

Carrot
Cassava/yuca root/manioc
Corn, organic, fresh or frozen
Ezekiel bread
Gluten-free bread
Gluten-free pasta
Legumes
Lentils
Oatmeal
Parsnips
Plantain
Potatoes
Pumpkin
Quinoa
Shirataki noodles
Sweet potatoes
Tapioca starch
Taro
Wild rice
Yam

FRUIT

Apples
Avocados
Bananas
Blackberries
Blueberries
Coconuts
Cherries
Cranberries
Dates
Figs
Grapefruit
Grapes
Honeydews
Kiwis
Lemons

Limes
Melons
Oranges
Peaches
Pears
Pineapples
Pomegranates
Raspberries
Strawberries

GOING FOR THE SUPER BURN

A Super Burn is just my clever little name for doing a longer Burn Zone to get *super* results. I'm sure you've heard of people who fast for twenty-four, thirty-six, or even forty-eight hours. Seems crazy, right? Why would you want to extend your Burn Zone? The longer you Burn, the better the results. "Fasting helps to correct hormone balance, and the benefits just get started at sixteen hours," says Dr. Jason Fung, author of *The Complete Guide to Fasting*. "When you fast for twenty-four hours, your body can actually burn up some of the loose skin on your body in a process called autophagy." Autophagy is a cellular process of recycling that your body can do to absorb old and unhealthy cells. It's this process that can "eat up" loose skin.

How to do a Super Burn: Pick a longer Burn Zone range. From twenty to twenty-four hours is best. If you get really hungry during the longer Burn time, it's fine to have Benefiber, a small handful of nuts, or another Burn Zone treat or beverage. These items won't trigger your blood sugar or your insulin, so you'll keep on burning fat. In fact, you'll be in such a strong fat-burning state that your body will use up any of that energy really quickly. My husband, Sam, and I have been amazed at how much our abs have slimmed down and become defined by making the Super Burn a regular part of our weekly routine.

Breaking a Super Burn: You want to be sure to transition gently from a longer Burn. There can be a temptation to overindulge after the Super Burn, but most Cruisers tell me that this is more of an emotional experience, not physical hunger. "I also encourage people not to eat in the middle of feeling really hungry," says Fung. "Hunger comes in waves that usually last about ten minutes. If you can ride it out, it will go away." Most Cruisers say that they naturally self-correct after a few days of adjusting to Cruise Control. That's because after a few days you'll have switched to being a fat-burning machine. Fat burners don't feel hungry—emotionally or physically—even after a Super Burn. When you are ready to break your Burn, have a handful of nuts and a glass of water. Wait for twenty to thirty minutes, and then go ahead and enjoy a feast. That's right, you can break a Super Burn with an abundant meal because your body is fully fasted and ready to accept a substantial amount of food—and to keep burning fat.

Congratulations on finishing your first twenty-eight days on Cruise Control. Well done. You now have all the tools for creating a lifetime of eating that will help you lose weight and maintain your new, slim figure. I'm so proud of you for completing your four weeks, but your work isn't done yet.

To make a sustainable change, I want you to make Cruise Control a lifestyle. You've already made a great start by sticking with Cruise Control for twenty-eight days. That's plenty of time for establishing new healthy and automated habits. Now you need to take it to the next level with high-octane recipes that will keep you full of energy and burning fat all day long. You've already automated a huge bunch of new healthy habits (it takes twenty-one days to create a habit). Now you just need to make it stick for life. In the next chapter, you'll find delicious recipes that keep you energized and burning fat for all your Zones. Keep reading.

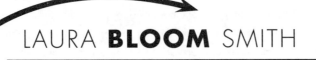

LAURA **BLOOM** SMITH

AGE: 50 | WEIGHT LOST: 50 POUNDS

What everyone needs to know: You'll learn how to nourish and respect your body. Well, that's what happened to me, and that's just a bonus in addition to so many other things, including dropping fifty pounds. I have high blood pressure and diabetes, and I am a breast cancer survivor. I had to go on several medications to manage my blood pressure and diabetes. I thought the old healthy me was history, but Cruise Control is a life-changing plan. I have seen such a dramatic change in my blood pressure that I've been able to reduce my medication, and my doctor has taken me entirely off of one of my diabetes meds. And the breast cancer? I have "no evidence of disease," just a year later. My disposition has changed from pessimist to optimist, I have more energy than ever before, and today I believe in myself and in my power to be the best driver to my best health. I will forever be grateful for this Cruise Control lifestyle! Don't miss out on the fabulous Cruiser support on the Cruise Control Facebook page.

CHAPTER 6

Recipes

Let food be your medicine.
—HIPPOCRATES

Welcome to what I'm betting will be your favorite part of Cruise Control: the recipes. I've spent the past two years elbows deep in food. Creating and crafting, adjusting and readjusting, and finally perfecting a whole bunch of delicious, satisfying, and easy-to-prepare meals and recipes that will not only be a pleasure to eat, but will have you burning fat, losing weight, and improving your health. It really wasn't a chore—taste testing was fun! You won't find ingredients that require you to travel to some small island out in the middle of the Atlantic—but you will find unique concoctions made from easy-to-find ingredients that I'm proud to share with you. I worked with thousands of my clients to curate and perfect the most delicious meals for the beginner cook as well as recipes that will satisfy and surprise an experienced chef. I've designed each section of recipes to progress from simple to more complex. All it takes is a well-stocked Cruise Control pantry (see shopping lists, beginning on page 91).

My family and I have happily and heartily eaten our way through this book more than once. Just a few tips before you dive in.

BE PREPARED

Before you start chopping, dicing, and preheating, take a minute to read through the entire recipe. Like, the whole thing. You'll get a big-picture understanding of what ingredients are involved, whether you have to prep anything in advance (like a sauce or vegetable), what tools you'll need, and how the dish is supposed to look when it's done.

UNDERSTAND SERVING SUGGESTIONS

The recipes I've included here stick to easy-to-find and simple-to-throw-together foods. I try to make these items easy to multiply for large families or to serve to just one or two people. The serving sizes are moderate. Listen to your own hunger and feelings of satisfaction. If a meal seems too big for you, then cut it down. If it doesn't seem substantial enough, bulk it up with some extra protein or healthy fat, or more vegetables. Many of my recipes are also great to take as leftovers for lunch on the following day. That way, you don't have to think about cooking every day. The rule of thumb is always to end your meal or snack feeling satisfied, *not* stuffed. Remember, while I don't want you to be "hangry," feeling some natural hunger before your next meal, or at the end of a Burn Zone, is healthy. It means that you've given your body the time it needs to do repair work, to burn fat, and to sharpen your mind. Try to embrace hunger as a positive sign that you are burning fat.

MY TOP CRUISE CONTROL TIPS

Use Cruise Control–Approved Ingredients

There are places in the book where we use ingredients like canned tomatoes, dressings, mustards, chicken broth, hot sauce, and so on. Though we don't specify this in each recipe, here is your friendly reminder to make sure all canned, bottled, frozen, or boxed foods mentioned follow Cruise Control guidelines. That means no added sugars, toxins, or bad fats, especially hydrogenated ones (see a full list of bad fats on page 58). I also highly recommend organic and local whenever possible. Read your labels! Do your homework.

Always Have a "Plan B"

There will be nights when the idea of making dinner seems about as likely as climbing Mount Everest. You will want to call for pizza, eat Goldfish or Teddy Grahams and drink wine, or maybe just curl up with a bowl of cereal and get back on track tomorrow. Don't! First things first. Make yourself a decaf cup of Cruise Control Coffee or Tea, take a ten-minute break, and breathe. Now turn to one of the following three "Plan B" items that can be prepped in under fifteen minutes, using the Cruise Control ingredients you'll already have on hand.

1. Mug Omelet, page 159

2. My Big Fat Greek Salad, page 166

3. Double Chocolate Fudge Mousse, page 151

Or feel free to come up with your own concoction using an approved protein, fat, and veggie or fruit. Maybe the My Big Fat Greek Salad (page 166) sounds good. Grab a sticky note and write "Plan B!" in big, bold letters and jot down the above three meals, or any three fast meals of your choice, and post them right on your fridge. A tough day doesn't have to ruin your healthy eating—ever! You're welcome.

Have Fun!

The kitchen is where you can get creative. Taking a variety of seemingly random ingredients, bringing them together, and making something delicious is just as inspired as painting a beautiful picture. At least that's how I look at it. When I take this perspective toward my cooking, it brings me happiness and serenity because I know that I'm creating something nourishing and substantial not only for myself but for the people I love. I encourage you to do the same. Get creative and improvise! Use spices and veggies you love and minimize those you don't like. Okay, we've talked enough here. Time to eat!

PABLO **GONZALEZ**

AGE: 42 | WEIGHT LOST: 25 POUNDS

What everyone needs to know: Don't throw away your skinny jeans before you try Cruise Control. I did. I'd thrown away all my "thin" clothes because I'd pretty much given up on losing weight and figured that I just had to accept that I was getting older, and getting bigger was merely part of it. My wife started on Cruise Control and, well, you know how that goes. She started talking about how great she was feeling, and then in two weeks, I could see that she was already losing weight and firming up at the same time! That convinced me to give the lifestyle a try, and now we're both dedicated Cruisers. Last week I found a suit that I hadn't worn since college. I hesitantly tried it on . . . and it fit! The best news is that I've not only changed physically. Cruise Control has impacted my entire outlook on life and what I am capable of doing to improve my health.

BURN ZONE BREAKFAST BEVERAGES

Cruise Control Coffee

In this recipe you can choose between MCT or coconut oil, and between grass-fed butter and ghee.

Servings: 1

1 cup (8 to 12 ounces) coffee
1 teaspoon to 2 tablespoons MCT oil or coconut oil
Pinch of Himalayan pink salt
1 to 2 tablespoons grass-fed, unsalted butter or grass-fed ghee

Place all of the ingredients in a blender and blend until creamy.

Note: If your mixture is really hot, be careful opening up the blender before you pour. I like to use my Blendtec blender because it seems to handle my coffee more safely (see "It's Better Blended," page 146). Also, remember that you can swap out coffee for tea. Finally, if you get hungry during your evening Burn Zone hours but don't want the caffeine, just make the recipe with any decaf beverage of your choice.

Cinnamon Spice Coffee

Servings: 1

1 cup (8 to 12 ounces) coffee
1 tablespoon MCT oil or coconut oil
¼ teaspoon ground cinnamon
1 tablespoon Cruise Control–friendly sweetener

Place all of the ingredients in a blender and blend until creamy.

Hot Coffee Cocoa

Servings: 1

1 cup (8 to 12 ounces) coffee
½ cup unsweetened almond milk
2 tablespoons coconut oil or MCT oil
2 tablespoons unsweetened cocoa powder
1 teaspoon pure vanilla extract
1 tablespoon Cruise Control–friendly sweetener
Whipped cream (optional)

1. Place the coffee, almond milk, oil, cocoa powder, vanilla, and sweetener in a blender and blend until creamy.

2. Top with whipped cream if desired.

Coconut Cream Latte

Servings: 1

1 cup (8 to 12 ounces) coffee
2 tablespoons unsweetened coconut milk
1 tablespoon MCT oil or coconut oil
1 tablespoon grass-fed, unsalted butter or grass-fed ghee
1 tablespoon Cruise Control–friendly sweetener

Place all of the ingredients in a blender and blend until creamy.

Iced Caffe Mocha

Servings: 1

2 tablespoons freshly ground coffee beans
¾ cup water
1 tablespoon grass-fed unsalted butter
1 to 2 teaspoons MCT oil
½ teaspoon pure vanilla extract
1 tablespoon Cruise Control–friendly sweetener
Ice, for serving

1. Brew the coffee using pour-over, automatic machine, or French press.

2. Pour the freshly brewed coffee, butter, oil, vanilla, and sweetener into a blender. Blend for 1 minute or until slightly frothy.

3. Serve over ice.

Iced Cruise Control Coffee

Servings: 1

1 cup (8 to 12 ounces) coffee
1 teaspoon to 2 tablespoons MCT or coconut oil
Pinch of Himalayan pink salt
1 to 2 tablespoons grass-fed, unsalted butter or grass-fed ghee
1 tablespoon Cruise Control–friendly sweetener
Ice, for serving*

1. Place the coffee, oil, salt, butter, and sweetener in a blender and blend until smooth and creamy.

2. Serve over ice.

*Note: If you have a powerful enough blender, this is super yummy with the ice blended with the other ingredients to make a Frappuccino-like drink (I use a Blendtec; see "It's Better Blended" below).

IT'S BETTER BLENDED

I've owned lots of blenders, and many powerful blenders, so trust me when I say that I think I've found the gold standard: Blendtec. I've never had one that works with the industrial power that this one does. Blendtec handles hot and cold items better than any other blender I've tried—I've yet to have the top pop off when blending hot, and ice cubes don't jam in it. It's great for making soups, drinks, sauces, condiments, and smoothies! For ordering information, see Resources, page 313.

Vanilla Cream Cold Brew

Servings: 1

8 ounces cold brew coffee
1 teaspoon pure vanilla extract
¼ cup heavy cream
1 teaspoon cinnamon, plus more for dusting
1½ cups unsweetened coconut milk
1 tablespoon Cruise Control–friendly sweetener
Whipped cream (optional)

1. Place the coffee, vanilla, cream, cinnamon, coconut milk, and sweetener in a blender and blend until creamy.

2. Top with whipped cream if desired and dust with cinnamon.

Fatty Iced Matcha Tea

Servings: 1

1 teaspoon matcha green tea powder
1 teaspoon grass-fed, unsalted butter or grass-fed ghee
2 teaspoons coconut oil
1 tablespoon Cruise Control–friendly sweetener
1 cup ice cubes
½ cup unsweetened coconut milk
1 teaspoon pure vanilla extract

1. In a small saucepan, heat ½ cup water over medium heat. Make sure water does not come to a boil.

2. Place the matcha powder in a small bowl and pour about 1 tablespoon of the hot water on top. Using a spoon, stir the matcha powder into a paste.

3. Combine the remainder of the hot water, ghee, coconut oil, sweetener, and matcha powder in a glass.

4. When the tea is mixed, add 1 cup crushed ice.

5. Combine coconut milk and vanilla and blend. Pour the mixture into the glass with the ice.

Vanilla Chai Tea Latte

Servings: 1

2 chai tea bags
1 tablespoon grass-fed, unsalted butter or grass-fed ghee
1 tablespoon MCT oil
½ teaspoon pure vanilla extract
1 tablespoon Cruise Control–friendly sweetener
Dash of cinnamon
2 tablespoons heavy cream

1. In a medium saucepan, bring 1½ cups water to a boil over medium-high heat. Add the tea bags and brew for 10 minutes. Remove the tea bags.

2. Blend the tea, butter, oil, vanilla, sweetener, cinnamon, and cream in a blender until creamy.

3. Pour into a cup and enjoy.

Butter Tea

Servings: 2

2 tablespoons regular or decaf loose-leaf black tea
¼ teaspoon salt
2 tablespoons grass-fed, unsalted butter
½ cup heavy cream

1. In a medium saucepan, bring 2 cups water to a boil over medium-high heat, then reduce the heat.

2. Add the tea to the water and simmer for 2 minutes, then strain.

3. Cool slightly, then add the salt, butter, and cream and whisk the mixture until frothy (for 30 seconds to 1 minute).

BURN ZONE TREATS

Double Chocolate Fudge Mousse

Servings: 2

Jell-O instant sugar-free chocolate pudding
2 cups heavy cream

1. Whisk the pudding mix with the cream in a medium bowl for 2 minutes.

2. Place the mixture in the refrigerator for 10 minutes to thicken and chill.

3. Pour the mousse into a glass or small bowl and enjoy!

Buttercup Gumdrops

Servings: 9

½ cup grass-fed, unsalted butter
1 cup coconut oil
¼ teaspoon sea salt
½ teaspoon cinnamon
1 tablespoon liquid stevia

1. Place the butter in a microwave-safe dish. Microwave on high for 30 to 45 seconds, until melted.

2. Combine the melted butter with the oil, sea salt, cinnamon, and stevia.

3. Whisk and pour into an ice cube tray.

4. Place the ice cube tray in the freezer for 4 hours.

5. Remove the ice cube tray from the freezer, pop out the gumdrops, and enjoy!

Vanilla Chia Seed Pudding

Servings: 6

½ cup chia seeds
One 14-ounce can full-fat coconut milk
2 teaspoons vanilla extract
⅓ cup Cruise Control–friendly sweetener

1. Mix the chia seeds with 1½ cups hot water in a large bowl.

2. Add coconut milk, vanilla, and sweetener and mix with a spoon.

3. Separate equally into 6 cups or bowls of your choice and refrigerate for 1 hour or overnight.

Peppermint Fat Bombs

Servings: 6

10 tablespoons coconut oil, melted
1 tablespoon Cruise Control–friendly sweetener
1 teaspoon peppermint extract
2 tablespoons unsweetened cocoa powder

1. Combine the coconut oil with the sweetener and peppermint extract in a small bowl.

2. Pour half of the mixture into ice cube trays. Place in the fridge. This will become the white layer.

3. Add cocoa powder to the remaining mixture, then pour on top of the white layer.

4. Place back into the refrigerator until set completely, then freeze for 2 to 3 hours.

Serve and enjoy!

Cinnamon Butter Bombs

Servings: 10

1 cup coconut butter
1 cup unsweetened coconut milk
1 teaspoon pure vanilla extract
½ teaspoon nutmeg
½ teaspoon cinnamon
1 teaspoon Cruise Control–friendly sweetener

1. Create a double boiler: Place a heat-proof glass bowl over a saucepan with a few inches of water in it.

2. Place all of the ingredients in a double boiler over medium heat.

3. Stir the ingredients as they melt.

4. When all the ingredients are combined, remove the bowl from the heat. (Careful—the bowl will be hot!)

5. Place the bowl in the refrigerator until the mixture solidifies.

6. Roll the mixture into 1-inch balls.

7. Place the bombs on a platter and refrigerate for 1 hour.

8. Serve and enjoy!

Strawberry Pops

Servings: 6

1 box sugar-free strawberry Jell-O
1 cup heavy cream

1. In a small saucepan, bring ½ cup water to a boil over medium-high heat. Remove from the heat.

2. Add the gelatin to the boiling water and mix until dissolved.

3. Pour the mixture into a blender and add the cream.

4. Blend until smooth.

5. Pour into popsicle molds and freeze for 4 hours.

6. Serve and enjoy!

BOOST ZONE MEALS

Zucchini "Linguine" Shakshuka

Servings: 1

1 tablespoon extra-virgin olive oil
½ onion, diced
1 clove garlic, crushed
½ red bell pepper, diced
1 can fire-roasted diced tomatoes
2 tablespoons tomato paste
2 cups zucchini in spiralized linguine-shaped noodles*
2 large eggs
1 sliced avocado
Salt and freshly ground pepper to taste (optional)

***Note**: A great time saver, I love to use a pack of Cece's Veggie Co. organic zucchini veggiccine. For more information, go to cecesveggieco. com. You can find many of Cece's vegetable noodles and riced veggies at grocery stores across the United States. Just hit the "where to buy" button on their website to find a market near you. Cece's veggies are perfect for Cruisers on the go who have no time for spiralizing or ricing their own veggies.

1. Preheat the oven to 350°F.

2. Heat oil in a cast-iron skillet for 3 to 4 minutes over medium-high heat. Add the onion, garlic, and bell pepper and sauté until starting to soften, about 3 minutes.

3. Drain a third of the liquid from the tomatoes and add the rest to the skillet with the tomato paste. Simmer for 2 to 3 more minutes.

4. Saving a small handful for garnish, stir in zucchini linguine and continue to cook for 3 more minutes.

5. Remove the skillet from the heat. Push the ingredients with a spoon to create two craters and crack the eggs into them.

6. Place the skillet in the preheated oven. Bake for 15 minutes or until the eggs are set.

7. Remove from the oven and top with avocado slices and raw zucchini linguine noodles. Season with salt and pepper if desired.

Dr. Weil's Tuscan Kale Salad

This is a great salad, jam-packed with powerful kale, that Dr. Andrew Weil shared with us from his restaurant, True Foods. It's also easy to throw together in a plastic container and take to work for lunch. We order it every time we go to Dr. Weil's restaurant.

Servings: 1

4 to 6 cups loosely packed, bite-size sliced leaves of Italian black
    kale, thick ribs removed
Juice of 1 lemon
3 to 4 tablespoons extra-virgin olive oil
2 cloves mashed garlic
Salt and freshly ground pepper to taste
Hot red pepper flakes to taste

⅔ cup grated Pecorino Toscano cheese or any other grated Italian cheese

½ cup freshly made breadcrumbs from lightly toasted bread

1. Place the kale in a serving bowl.

2. Whisk together the lemon juice, olive oil, garlic, salt, black pepper, and a generous pinch of red pepper flakes.

3. Pour the dressing over the kale and toss well. Add the cheese, reserving 2 tablespoons, and toss again.

4. Let the kale sit for at least 5 minutes.

5. Add the breadcrumbs, toss again, and top with the remaining cheese.

Mug Omelet

If I arrive home starving, I'll often throw this super simple "omelet" together. I love breakfast for dinner. You can also substitute any leftover cooked protein for the ham, and kale or other greens for the spinach.

Servings: 1

2 large eggs
½ bell pepper, diced
2 slices ham, diced
¼ cup fresh spinach
Salt and freshly ground black pepper to taste

1. Combine all of the ingredients in a microwavable mug.

2. Cook for 2 to 3 minutes, making sure the egg doesn't bubble over. Stir halfway through the cooking process.

3. Enjoy!

One-Pan Italian Sausage & Veggies

Servings: 6

2 cups carrot
2 cups red potato
2⅓ cups zucchini
2 cups red bell pepper
1½ cups broccoli
16 ounces smoked Italian turkey or chicken sausage
1½ teaspoons dried basil
1½ teaspoons dried oregano
1½ teaspoons dried parsley
1½ teaspoons garlic powder
½ teaspoon onion powder
½ teaspoon dried thyme
½ teaspoon salt (if desired)
⅛ teaspoon freshly ground black pepper (optional)
4½ tablespoons extra-virgin olive oil
⅛ teaspoon crushed red pepper flakes (optional)
⅓ cup freshly grated Parmesan cheese (optional)
Fresh parsley (optional)

1. Preheat the oven to 400°F. Line a large rimmed baking sheet with parchment paper or foil.

2. Peel and thinly slice the carrots. Wash and chop the potatoes in half, then cut each half into 10 to 12 pieces.

3. Cut the zucchini in half and cut each side into thick coins. Coarsely chop the broccoli. Remove the stems and seeds from the bell peppers and chop into medium-size pieces. Chop the sausage into thick coins.

4. Arrange the veggies and sausage on the prepared baking sheet.

5. In a small bowl combine the basil, oregano, parsley, garlic powder, onion powder, thyme, crushed red pepper flakes, and salt and pepper if desired with the olive oil. Stir to combine.

6. Pour the seasoning-and-oil mixture on top of the veggies and sausage and toss to coat.

7. Place in the oven and cook for 15 minutes. Remove from the oven, toss the veggies and sausage, and return to the oven for another 10 to 20 minutes or until the vegetables are crisp-tender.

8. Top with freshly grated Parmesan cheese and parsley if desired.

9. Serve and enjoy!

One-Pot Shrimp Alfredo

Servings: 4

1 tablespoon grass-fed salted butter
1 pound raw shrimp
4 ounces cream cheese, cubed
½ cup whole milk
1 tablespoon garlic powder
1 teaspoon dried basil
1 teaspoon salt
½ cup shredded Parmesan cheese
5 whole sun-dried tomatoes, cut into strips
¼ cup baby kale or spinach

1. Melt the butter in a large skillet over medium heat.

2. Add the shrimp to the skillet and reduce the heat to medium-low.

3. Turn shrimp after 30 seconds and cook the other side until slightly pink. This is important because the sauce will continue to cook the shrimp once it is added. If you overcook the shrimp, it will become tough and rubbery!

4. Add the cream cheese cubes and milk to the pan and reduce the heat to medium. Stir frequently until the cream cheese has melted into the milk and there are no lumps.

5. Sprinkle with the garlic powder, basil, and salt and stir well.

6. Add the Parmesan and stir to combine. Let simmer until the sauce begins to thicken.

7. Complete the dish by folding in the sun-dried tomatoes and baby kale.

8. Remove from the heat and serve.

Bruschetta Burgers

Servings: 4

1 pound ground chicken
¼ cup grated Parmesan cheese
2 cloves garlic
1 teaspoon onion powder
2 tablespoons torn basil leaves, plus more for garnish
½ tablespoon balsamic vinegar
Kosher salt
Freshly ground black pepper
1 tablespoon extra-virgin olive oil
5 thick slices fresh mozzarella
8 slices tomato
1 cup baby spinach
Balsamic glaze, for drizzling

1. In a large bowl, combine the ground chicken, Parmesan, garlic, onion powder, basil, and vinegar. Season with salt and pepper, then form the mixture into 4 small patties, depending on the size of your tomatoes. (They should be approximately the same size!)

2. In a large skillet, heat the olive oil over medium heat. Add the patties and turn after 6 minutes and seared on one side. Flip again for about 4 minutes, then top with the mozzarella. Cover the skillet and cook for 2 to 3 more minutes, until the cheese melts and the chicken is cooked through.

3. Slice the tomatoes in half. Season the bottom tomato halves with salt and pepper. Top with the baby spinach, the burgers, and the basil garnish, then drizzle with the balsamic glaze. Top with the remaining tomato halves.

Taco-Stuffed Avocados

Servings: 6

1 pound ground beef
1 tablespoon chili powder
½ teaspoon salt
¾ teaspoon cumin
½ teaspoon dried oregano
¼ teaspoon garlic powder
¼ teaspoon onion powder
4 ounces tomato sauce
3 avocados, halved
1 cup shredded Cheddar cheese
¼ cup cherry tomatoes, sliced
¼ cup lettuce, shredded
6 tablespoons sour cream
⅓ cup cilantro, chopped

1. Add the ground beef to a medium saucepan. Cook over medium heat until browned.

2. Drain the grease and add the chili powder, salt, cumin, oregano, garlic powder, onion powder, and tomato sauce. Stir to combine and cook for 3 to 4 minutes.

3. Remove the pits from halved avocados and fill with the taco meat. Top each "taco" with cheese, tomatoes, one tablespoon of sour cream, and a sprinkling of cilantro.

4. Serve and enjoy!

Portobello Mini Pizzas

This is a Cruiser favorite. The Facebook Cruise Control community raves about this little pizza.

Servings: 2

2 large portobello caps, stems removed
½ cup pesto
1 cup shredded Italian blend cheese
10 black kalamata olives
1 tablespoon capers
Pinch of crushed red pepper flakes and basil for garnish (optional)

1. Preheat the oven to 375°F. Place the mushrooms on a rimmed baking sheet. Spread ¼ cup pesto in each mushroom cap.

2. Fill the centers with cheese, then top with olives and capers.

3. Bake for 10 to 15 minutes or just until the cheese is bubbly and mushrooms are starting to soften.

4. Sprinkle with red pepper flakes and basil, if using, or refrigerate for up to a day and reheat before serving.

My Big Fat Greek Salad

This is my go-to lunch. When I'm traveling, I carry the salad in one container and the dressing in another. It is also easy to order in restaurants that serve Greek salads. I just bring my own dressing, or carry one of the FBOMB MCT oils (see "Drop an FBOMB," page 58) and ask your server for vinegar.

Servings: 2

Salad

    2 medium skinless, boneless chicken breasts, pounded flat
    1 tablespoon extra-virgin olive oil
    1½ teaspoons dried oregano
    1 garlic clove, crushed
    Salt and freshly ground pepper to taste
    2 cups romaine lettuce, chopped
    1 avocado, peeled, pitted, and chopped
    1 cup cherry or grape tomatoes, cut in half
    ½ red onion, sliced thinly
    One 6.5-ounce jar diced marinated artichoke hearts
    ¼ cup feta cheese
    ¼ cup pitted kalamata olives

Dressing

    ¼ cup extra-virgin olive oil
    2 tablespoons raw apple cider vinegar
    Juice of ½ lemon
    1 small garlic clove, minced
    ½ teaspoon Dijon mustard
    ½ teaspoon dried oregano
    ½ teaspoon salt
    ½ teaspoon freshly ground black pepper

1. Pound the chicken flat with a meat tenderizer or slice the chicken breasts in half to make thinner.

2. In a medium bowl or Ziploc bag, combine the chicken, olive oil, oregano, garlic, salt, and pepper.

3. Heat a large, heavy-duty pan over medium heat and cook each side of chicken for 5 to 6 minutes or until tender and cooked through.

4. Remove the chicken from the pan, cool for 5 minutes, then slice or chop.

5. Combine all of the ingredients for the dressing in a small bowl and whisk.

6. In a large bowl, combine the lettuce, avocado, tomatoes, onion, artichoke hearts, feta, and olives. Top with chicken and drizzle the dressing generously.

No-Cook Bento Box

Okay, so you might not have an actual bento box lying around, but you can use any rectangular-shaped plastic container to pack this handy meal for your lunch.

Servings: 1

2 tablespoons cream cheese
1 teaspoon ranch seasoning
3 slices deli turkey with no added sugar
½ small cucumber, sliced
½ red bell pepper, sliced
¼ cup blackberries
¼ cup Colby Jack cheese or Cheddar cheese, cubed
¼ cup hazelnuts

1. In a small bowl, mix the cream cheese and ranch seasoning until smooth. Smear the cream cheese mixture on the turkey slices. Top with a slice of cucumber and bell pepper, and then roll up in the turkey and cut in half.

2. Place the turkey roll-ups in the container with the blackberries, cheese, and nuts.

3. Enjoy!

Egg Drop Soup

Servings: 6

2 quarts chicken or bone broth (Kettle & Fire)*
1 tablespoon freshly grated turmeric or 1 teaspoon ground turmeric
1 tablespoon freshly grated ginger or 1 teaspoon ground ginger
2 cloves garlic, minced
1 small chili pepper, sliced
2 cups sliced brown mushrooms
2 tablespoons coconut aminos or soy sauce
4 cups chopped Swiss chard leaves or spinach
4 large eggs
2 medium spring onions, sliced
2 tablespoons freshly chopped cilantro
1 teaspoon salt or to taste
6 tablespoons extra-virgin olive oil

*You can find many great recipes for bone broth online. These are wonderful, but they are time-consuming—like hours of time, if not overnight—and they can leave your kitchen smelling like beef. My go-to bone broth is Kettle & Fire; see kettleandfire.com. They make their broth with all natural ingredients, they do the slow-cooking for you, and their broth is vacuum packed and has a two-year shelf life.

1. Pour the chicken stock in a large pot and place over medium heat, until it starts to simmer.

2. Add the turmeric, ginger, garlic, chili pepper, mushrooms, and coconut aminos to the stock and simmer for 5 minutes.

3. Add the chard leaves and cook for 1 minute. In a separate bowl, whisk the eggs and slowly pour them into the simmering soup.

4. Keep stirring until the eggs are cooked, then remove the pot from the heat. Add the onions and cilantro to the soup and season with salt and pepper.

5. Pour into a serving bowl and drizzle with the olive oil. Eat immediately or let it cool down and store in an airtight container for up to 5 days.

BLT Ranch Wrap

Servings: 1

Ranch Dressing
    1 tablespoon mayonnaise
    1 teaspoon lemon juice
    1 teaspoon dried parsley
    ¼ teaspoon garlic powder
    ¼ teaspoon onion powder
    Pinch of sea salt and freshly ground black pepper

Lettuce Wrap
    3 to 4 leaves leaf lettuce
    2 slices cooked bacon
    2 to 3 tomatoes, sliced
    ¼ small avocado, sliced

1. Mix the ranch ingredients together in a small bowl.

2. Arrange the lettuce in a single layer slightly overlapping. Drizzle with ranch dressing.

3. Top with bacon, tomato, and avocado.

4. Roll the lettuce like a sushi roll and tuck the edges as you go. Once wrapped, cut in half.

5. Enjoy!

Zoodle Spaghetti & Meatballs

This is a great one for kids. We make it every Monday for my boys.

Servings: 6

Meatballs
    ¾ pound ground beef
    ½ pound ground turkey
    ¼ cup grated Parmesan cheese
    1 teaspoon Italian seasoning
    Salt and freshly ground black pepper to taste
    ¼ onion, minced
    2 garlic cloves, minced
    2 large eggs
    ¼ cup whole milk
    2 tablespoons gluten-free breadcrumbs
    2 tablespoons chopped fresh parsley
    Extra-virgin olive oil

Sauce and Zoodles
    5 to 6 medium zucchini, about 2¼ pounds total
    4-5 tablespoons extra-virgin olive oil
    1 medium onion, finely chopped
    2 carrots, peeled and diced
    3 cloves garlic, finely chopped
    3 tablespoons tomato paste
    One 14.5-ounce can diced tomatoes
    One 14.5-ounce can crushed tomatoes
    1 cup low-sodium beef broth
    1 teaspoon dried oregano
    1 bay leaf
    ¾ teaspoon dried basil
    Chopped fresh parsley, for serving
    Grated Parmesan cheese, for serving

1. For the meatballs: Combine ground beef, turkey, cheese, Italian seasoning, salt, pepper, onion, and garlic together. Mix in eggs, milk, breadcrumbs, and parsley until just combined.

2. Form meatballs and cook in 2 to 3 tablespoons of oil over medium heat for 8 to 10 minutes.

3. For the sauce: Heat 1 tablespoon olive oil in a wide, deep skillet on medium-high heat and add onion and carrots. Sauté for 2 to 3 minutes.

4. Add garlic and tomato paste and mix in onion, carrot mixture. Add both cans of tomatoes, the broth, oregano, bay leaf, and basil. Cover and turn heat to low. Simmer for 20 to 30 minutes, stirring occasionally.

5. For the zoodles: Spiralize the zucchini into zucchini noodles using a spiralizer or vegetable peeler. Add the olive oil to a pan and cook the zoodles over medium heat for 1 to 2 minutes or until slightly softened and beginning to brown.

6. Transfer the zoodles and meatballs to a serving bowl. Then add the sauce and sprinkling of freshly chopped parsley and Parmesan cheese.

Nacho Steak Skillet

Servings: 6

1½ pounds cauliflower
⅓ cup coconut oil
1 teaspoon chili powder
½ teaspoon turmeric
Salt and freshly ground black pepper to taste
8 ounces beef. Any boneless cut steak on the thinner side will do, such as strip, rib-eye, or flat iron
1 tablespoon butter
¼ cup shredded Cheddar cheese

¼ cup shredded Monterey Jack cheese
⅛ cup canned jalapeño slices
⅓ cup sour cream
1 avocado
½ teaspoon hot sauce

1. Preheat the oven to 400°F. Remove the leaves and bottom of the stem from the cauliflower. Slice the cauliflower across the head.

2. In a large bowl combine the coconut oil, chili powder, and turmeric. Add the cauliflower and toss until it's evenly coated.

3. Spread the cauliflower out on a rimmed baking sheet. Season with salt and pepper. Roast for 20 to 25 minutes, until it has softened and the edges are golden brown.

4. Preheat a cast-iron skillet over medium-high heat. Season both sides of the steak with salt and pepper. Melt the butter in the skillet. Add the steak. Cook through, about 3 minutes, then flip to cook the other side for 3 more minutes. Remove the steak from the pan.

5. Allow the steak to rest for 5 to 10 minutes.

6. Once the cauliflower is done, remove it from the oven and transfer the florets to the cast-iron skillet.

7. Slice up the steak into strips.

8. Top the cauliflower with the steak. Then top with both shredded cheeses and the jalapeño slices. Place the skillet in the oven and bake for another 5 to 10 minutes, until the cheese has melted.

9. Peel and de-pit the avocado and mash it in a small bowl with the hot sauce.

10. Serve with sour cream, guacamole, and hot sauce.

Cashew Chicken

Servings: 3

¼ cup raw cashews
3 skinless, boneless chicken thighs
½ medium green bell pepper
¼ medium white onion
2 tablespoons coconut oil
1 tablespoon green onions
1 tablespoon minced garlic
1½ teaspoons chili garlic sauce
½ teaspoon ground ginger
Salt and freshly ground black pepper to taste
1 tablespoon rice wine vinegar
1 tablespoon sesame oil
1 teaspoon sesame seeds

1. Heat a medium pan over low heat and toast the cashews for 8 minutes. Remove and set aside.

2. Dice the chicken thighs into chunks. Cut the bell pepper and white onion into large chunks.

3. Raise the heat to high and add the coconut oil to the pan.

4. Add the chicken and cook for 5 minutes.

5. Add the bell pepper, white onions, green onions, garlic, chili garlic sauce, ginger, salt, and black pepper. Cook for 2 to 3 minutes.

6. Add the rice wine vinegar and cashews. Cook for 2 to 3 more minutes.

7. Serve in a bowl. Top with sesame seeds and drizzle with sesame oil.

8. Enjoy!

Ham & Goat Cheese Frittata

Servings: 6

1 tablespoon extra-virgin olive oil
¼ onion, diced
½ pound asparagus, ends trimmed and cut into approximately
   2-inch pieces
⅓ cup chopped broccoli florets
½ red bell pepper, chopped
8 large eggs
¼ cup heavy cream
6 ounces chopped smoked ham
½ teaspoon garlic powder
½ cup grated Cheddar cheese
4 ounces goat cheese

1. Preheat the oven to 400°F.

2. In an oven-proof nonstick skillet over medium heat, heat the olive oil and add the onion, asparagus, broccoli, and bell pepper. Cook for 2 to 3 minutes.

3. Whisk eggs with the cream and ham. Stir in the garlic powder and Cheddar cheese. Pour the eggs into the same pan with the asparagus, and top with crumbled goat cheese.

4. Transfer the pan to the oven and cook for 15 minutes.

5. Cut into wedges and serve!

Broccoli Cheese Soup

Servings: 8

2 tablespoons grass-fed salted butter
1 stalk celery, chopped
1 onion, chopped
1½ pounds broccoli florets, chopped
3 cups chicken broth or bone broth
1 teaspoon garlic powder
1 teaspoon paprika
Salt and freshly ground black pepper to taste
3 cups Cheddar cheese, grated
1 pouch Parmesan crisps (Parm Crisps)*

1. In a stockpot, melt the butter over medium heat. Cook the celery and onion in the butter until softened, about 3 minutes. Stir in the broccoli, then cover with the stock. Simmer for 10 minutes.

2. Reduce the heat and stir in the garlic powder and paprika and salt and pepper if desired. Add the Cheddar cheese gradually and continue to stir until melted.

3. Top with Parm Crisps.*

4. Serve and enjoy.

*Note: Parm Crisps are yummy chips made from real cheese and other natural ingredients, and you can find them on parmcrisps.com or at Amazon. You can use original or jalapeño (if you want a kick) as your soup topping. I've become a bit of a cheesehead because of these zero-carb healthy fats. I love to put these on salads and soups, and I definitely love them for a quick snack. Just be careful! Parm Crisps are highly addictive.

5-Minute Tuna Salad

Servings: 2

¼ cup mayonnaise
1 tablespoon lemon juice
2 tablespoons extra-virgin olive oil
1 tablespoon chopped parsley
¼ teaspoon salt
¼ teaspoon freshly ground black pepper
1 head romaine lettuce
1 medium cucumber, sliced
½ small onion, sliced
One 5-ounce can tuna, drained
8 large olives, sliced
4 large hard-boiled eggs

1. Place the mayonnaise, lemon juice, olive oil, parsley, salt, and pepper in a small bowl and whisk until blended.

2. Separate the lettuce leaves and fold them into a medium bowl.

3. Add the cucumber, onion, tuna, and olives on top of the lettuce leaves.

4. Slice the eggs into quarters and add to salad.

5. Drizzle the dressing onto the salad.

6. Serve and enjoy!

Sheet Pan Salmon & Asparagus

Servings: 4

1 pound wild-caught salmon fillets
2 tablespoons mayonnaise
1 teaspoon Dijon mustard
¼ cup grated Parmesan cheese
1 pound fresh asparagus, ends trimmed
1 tablespoon extra-virgin olive oil
2 lemons
½ teaspoon kosher salt
¼ teaspoon ground black pepper
2 tablespoons chopped parsley, for garnish

1. Preheat the oven to 325°F.

2. Rinse and pat dry the salmon fillets; remove any bones.

3. Mix together the mayonnaise and mustard in a small bowl.

4. Brush the mayonnaise mixture over the top of the salmon.

5. Sprinkle the Parmesan on top.

6. Place the asparagus on a rimmed baking sheet and drizzle with olive oil.

7. Spread the asparagus out on the baking sheet, leaving room in the center for the salmon.

8. Place the salmon on the baking sheet.

9. Cut the lemons in half and place them, cut-side up, on the baking sheet.

10. Sprinkle the entire pan with salt and pepper.

11. Bake for 18 minutes. Remove from the oven and squeeze lemon juice over the asparagus and salmon, removing any lemon seeds.

12. Garnish with parsley and serve warm.

Cauliflower Pepperoni Pizza

Servings: 2

Crust
   1½ cup cauliflower rice
   1 large egg
   ½ cup grated mozzarella cheese
   ⅓ cup grated Parmesan cheese
   1 teaspoon dried basil
   1 teaspoon dried oregano
   ½ teaspoon garlic powder
   ½ teaspoon salt
   Extra-virgin olive oil

Sauce
   1 clove garlic, minced
   1 tablespoon fresh basil
   1 tablespoon tomato puree
   2 tablespoons extra-virgin olive oil
   ½ teaspoon dried fennel seeds
   1 tablespoon fresh parsley

Toppings
   ¼ cup grated mozzarella cheese
   10 slices pepperoni ham
   ¼ cup chopped fresh basil leaves
   ¼ cup grated Parmesan cheese

1. Preheat the oven to 450°F.

2. In a large bowl, mix the cauliflower rice with the egg, mozzarella, Parmesan, basil, oregano, garlic powder, and salt.

3. Line a baking sheet with a nonstick spray or parchment paper. Press the cauliflower mixture evenly on the pan. Spray with some extra-virgin olive oil.

4. Bake for 15 to 20 minutes, until the mixture begins to turn golden brown. Remove the baking sheet from the oven and set aside.

5. For the pizza sauce, mash the garlic and chop the basil. Place them in a small bowl and add the tomato puree, olive oil, fennel seeds, and parsley. Mix with a spoon.

6. Spread the sauce evenly over the pizza crust. Top with grated mozzarella, pepperoni ham, basil, and Parmesan.

7. Place in the oven and cook for an additional 10 minutes.

8. Serve and enjoy!

BOOST ZONE SNACKS

Crispy Avocado Fries

Servings: 4

Cooking spray, for greasing the baking sheet and spraying the avocado wedges
2 firm avocados, cut into ½-inch wedges
½ teaspoon salt
¼ teaspoon freshly ground black pepper
⅓ cup white whole-wheat flour
2 large eggs
1 cup whole-wheat panko breadcrumbs
⅓ cup mayonnaise
2 tablespoons Sriracha

1. Preheat the oven to 425°F.

2. Spray a rimmed baking sheet with cooking spray.

3. Season the avocados with salt and pepper. Place the flour, eggs, and panko in 3 separate dishes. Coat the avocado wedges in the flour, then dip in the egg. Coat both sides with the panko.

4. Place the wedges on the prepared baking sheet. Coat both sides with cooking spray.

5. Bake for 30 minutes. Flip the wedges halfway through.

6. Whisk the mayonnaise and Sriracha in a small bowl.

7. Serve the avocado fries with the aioli and enjoy!

Bacon Guac Bombs

Servings: 6

4 large slices bacon
½ large avocado
¼ cup unsalted, grass-fed butter
1 small chili pepper, chopped
2 cloves garlic, crushed
1 to 2 tablespoons freshly chopped cilantro
1 tablespoon fresh lime juice
¼ teaspoon salt
Freshly ground black pepper
½ small white onion, diced

1. Preheat the oven to 375°F.

2. Line a rimmed baking sheet with parchment paper. Lay the bacon strips out flat. Place the baking sheet in the oven and cook for about 15 minutes, until the bacon is golden brown.

3. Halve, de-seed, and peel the avocado. Place the avocado, butter, chili pepper, garlic, cilantro, and lime juice in a bowl and season with salt and pepper.

4. Mash until well combined. Add the diced onion and mix well. Place in the refrigerator for 10 minutes.

5. Crumble the bacon into small pieces. Remove the guacamole mixture from the fridge and scoop out 6 balls.

6. Roll each ball in the bacon crumbles and place on a dish.

7. Serve and enjoy!

Cabbage Chips

Servings: 6

1 large head cabbage
¼ cup grated Parmesan cheese
2 teaspoons extra-virgin olive oil
Kosher salt
Freshly ground black pepper

1. Preheat the oven to 250°F. Set 2 wire racks inside 2 rimmed baking sheets. Tear the cabbage leaves into large pieces, leaving out the thickest part of the ribs.

2. Toss the cabbage leaves with the Parmesan and olive oil, then season with salt and pepper.

3. Arrange in a single layer on wire racks.

4. Bake for 35 minutes or until golden and crispy.

5. Serve and enjoy!

Broccoli Cheesy Bread

Servings: 8

3 cups broccoli, riced
1 large egg
1½ cups shredded mozzarella
¼ cup Parmesan cheese, grated
2 cloves garlic, minced
½ teaspoon dried oregano
Kosher salt
Freshly ground black pepper

1. Preheat the oven to 425°F and line a large rimmed baking sheet with parchment paper.

2. Place the riced broccoli in a large microwave-safe bowl. Microwave, covered for 1 minute to steam. Ring out the moisture from the broccoli using a paper towel.

3. Transfer the broccoli to a large bowl and add the egg, 1 cup mozzarella, the Parmesan, and the garlic. Season with the oregano, salt, and pepper. Transfer the dough to the prepared baking sheet and shape into a thin, round crust.

4. Bake for 20 minutes or until golden. Top with remaining ½ cup mozzarella and bake for 10 more minutes or until the cheese is melted and the crust is crispy.

5. Serve and enjoy!

Pizza Chips

I like to use Applegate turkey pepperoni because they don't add nitrates and are gluten-free.

Servings: 7

6 ounces sliced pepperoni
1½ cups mozzarella cheese, shredded

1. Preheat the oven to 400°F.

2. On a rimmed baking sheet, arrange the pepperoni slices in batches of 4, close together.

3. Bake for 5 minutes. Sprinkle the cheese on top. Bake for another 3 minutes, or until the cheese is melted and crisp.

4. Place the chips on paper towels. Let cool for 5 minutes.

5. Serve and enjoy!

Celery Cream Cheese Boat

My acting clients love these treats because they are easy to have on set and make a substantial and perfect on-the-go snack.

Servings: 4

10 stalks celery, rinsed
Two 1-ounce packages cream cheese
1 teaspoon everything bagel seasoning

1. Cut the celery stalks into 3 sections each.

2. Stuff the celery with the cream cheese.

3. Sprinkle the stalks with everything bagel seasoning.

4. Serve and enjoy!

Super Trail Mix

Servings: 6

½ cup almond slices
½ cup whole almonds, raw
½ cup pecan halves
½ cup walnut pieces
½ cup coconut flakes, unsweetened
¼ cup chia seeds
¼ cup flaxseeds
½ cup coconut oil, melted
1 tablespoon ground cinnamon
1 teaspoon Himalayan pink salt
¼ cup Cruise Control–friendly sweetener

1. Preheat the oven to 350°F. Line a rimmed baking sheet with parchment paper.

2. In a large bowl, combine the sliced almonds, whole almonds, pecans, walnuts, coconut flakes, chia seeds, and flaxseeds.

3. Add the coconut oil to the mix.

4. Sprinkle in the cinnamon and salt. Mix well.

5. Place the mixture on the prepared baking sheet and bake for 15 minutes.

6. Let the trail mix cool for 30 minutes.

7. Sprinkle with the Cruise Control–friendly sweetener, serve, and enjoy.

Cauliflower Cheese Muffins

Servings: 8

Nonstick cooking spray, for greasing the muffin pan
1 large cauliflower, chopped
1 cup heavy cream
2 ounces cream cheese
½ teaspoon onion powder
Freshly ground black pepper to taste
1¾ cups shredded sharp Cheddar cheese
2 large eggs, beaten

1. Preheat the oven to 350°F. Spray a muffin tin with nonstick spray.

2. Bring a large pot of water to a boil over medium-high heat. Add the cauliflower and boil until tender, about 7 to 10 minutes. Drain.

3. Cook the cream and cream cheese in a medium saucepan over low heat until creamy, about 5 minutes, stirring constantly. Add the onion powder and pepper.

4. Add 1 cup shredded Cheddar, the eggs, and the cauliflower to the mixture and stir until smooth.

5. Spoon into the prepared muffin tin and sprinkle with the remaining ¾ cup shredded Cheddar and bake for 20 minutes.

6. Cool for 15 minutes before removing from the muffin pan.

7. Serve and enjoy!

BOOST ZONE DESSERTS

Chocolate Salted Peanut Butter Cups

Servings: 6

Chocolate Coating
- 6 tablespoons coconut oil, melted
- 6 tablespoons unsweetened cocoa powder
- 3 tablespoons Swerve Confectioner's sweetener

Peanut Butter Filling
- 2 tablespoons cocoa butter, melted
- 2 teaspoons no-sugar-added peanut butter
- 1 tablespoon Swerve Confectioner's sweetener
- ½ teaspoon kosher salt or sea salt

1. Place muffin liners in 6 cups of a muffin tin. Set aside.

2. Whisk together the coconut oil, cocoa powder, and Swerve in a medium bowl. Place a tablespoon of chocolate mixture in each muffin liner. Place in the freezer for 5 minutes.

3. In a separate, microwave-safe bowl, whisk together the cocoa butter, peanut butter, Swerve, and salt. Once combined, microwave on high for 10 seconds. Remove the chocolate from the freezer and add 1½ teaspoons of the peanut butter mixture to the frozen chocolate coating. Return to the freezer for another 3 minutes.

4. Remove from the freezer and add 1 tablespoon of the remaining chocolate in each cup, covering the peanut butter mixture. Freeze again for 5 minutes. Then eat and enjoy.

5. Store in fridge or freezer in an airtight storage container. If desired, let soften for 15 to 20 minutes before eating.

Snap Cookie Ice-Cream Slider

Servings: 6

6 ounces low-sugar or nondairy ice cream
12 Keto-Snap cookies (see "My Favorite Cookie," the following page)

1. Place about 2 tablespoons of ice cream on the bottom of a cookie and spread to the edge. Top with another cookie.

2. Repeat to make 6 ice-cream sliders.

3. Serve and enjoy!

MY FAVORITE COOKIE

I love these little Keto-Snap cookies. With a tip of the hat to Dr. Seuss, I love them at night, and I love them on flights. I love them in my car, and I've shared them with some stars. They are made with healthy and natural ingredients and make a great little snack when that sweet tooth is calling. Plus, they are perfect for dipping into a cup of coffee or tea for an afternoon pick-me-up. They are lightly sweet, crisp and crunchy, and made with cinnamon. My boys and I love to top these cookies with whipped cream for an extra decadent Boost Zone dessert. And the best news about these guys, besides the fact that your kids will love them? They won't spike your blood sugar dangerously or signal insulin to store calories as fat, so you can enjoy these guilt-free anytime you feel a craving for sweets. You can have three cookies, and only 3 percent of that will be carbohydrate, but you'll get a nice 5 grams of protein and 3 grams of fiber. Confession: I usually can't stop at three! For more information, see Resources, page 304.

Chocolate Avocado Pops

Servings: 10

3 ripe avocados
⅓ cup lime juice
3 tablespoons Cruise Control–friendly sweetener
¾ cup coconut milk
1 cup dark chocolate chips (55% cocoa)
1 tablespoon coconut oil

1. In the bowl of a blender, combine avocados, lime juice, sweetener, and coconut milk. Blend until smooth and pour into popsicle molds.

2. Freeze for 6 hours or overnight, until the molds are firm.

3. In a medium microwave-safe bowl, combine the dark chocolate chips and coconut oil. Microwave until melted, then let cool to room temperature.

4. Dunk the frozen pops in the chocolate and serve.

Chocolate Pudding

Servings: 2

1 large, overripe avocado
2 ounces plain full-fat triple-cream yogurt (Peak Yogurt)*
¼ cup unsweetened cocoa powder
¼ cup Cruise Control–friendly sweetener
1½ teaspoons cinnamon
¼ teaspoon cayenne pepper
¼ teaspoon pure vanilla extract

1. Place all of the ingredients in a blender and process until smooth.

2. Spoon into 2 bowls and enjoy!

   *Note: You can use other whole-fat plain yogurts, but I like Peak Yogurt because it is designed to be lower in sugar, so more Cruise Control–friendly. It's also sooo super creamy. This is a great on-the-go dessert and makes a great savory dip for veggies. If you find that you are a little low on your fat intake, you can use this yogurt for a quick and healthy boost. You can find it at peakyogurt.com.

Million-Dollar Milkshake

This is my adaptation of my favorite smoothie in Malibu at a place called SunLife Organics. If any Cruisers are ever in Malibu, I highly recommend stopping by for a similar treat. You won't regret it.

Servings: 1

½ cup unsweetened almond milk
1 tablespoon raw cashew butter
1 scoop grass-fed vanilla whey protein
1 teaspoon raw cacao powder
1 teaspoon chia seeds
1 tablespoon MCT oil
1 tablespoon Cruise Control–friendly sweetener

Place all of the ingredients in a blender and blend until and smooth.

Chocolate Macadamia Nut Parfait

Servings: 1

5 ounces plain full-fat triple-cream yogurt
One 1-ounce packet of FBOMB Salted Chocolate Macadamia Nut
    Butter
2 tablespoons macadamia nuts

1. Open a 5-ounce container of natural, full-fat yogurt and squeeze a packet of FBOMB Salted Chocolate Macadamia Nut Butter into it.

2. Stir and top with macadamia nuts.

3. Serve and enjoy!

Almond Butter Cookies

Servings: 15

1 cup natural almond butter
½ cup Cruise Control–friendly sweetener
1 large egg
1 teaspoon pure vanilla extract
¼ teaspoon sea salt
½ teaspoon ground cinnamon

1. Preheat the oven to 350°F. Line a baking sheet with parchment paper.

2. In a large bowl, mix together the almond butter and sweetener until smooth. Mix in the egg, vanilla, salt, and cinnamon and stir until well combined.

3. Scoop into 15 cookies.

4. Place the dough balls on the prepared baking sheet 2 inches apart, and then use a fork to flatten them and form a crisscross pattern.

5. Bake for 12 minutes or until the cookies are slightly browned on the bottom.

6. Cool on the baking sheet for 3 minutes.

7. Serve and enjoy!

Double Fudge Brownies

Servings: 16

Nonstick cooking spray, for greasing the pan
½ cup unsalted grass-fed butter, melted
⅔ cup Cruise Control–friendly sweetener
3 large eggs
½ teaspoon pure vanilla extract
½ cup almond flour
⅓ cup cocoa powder
1 tablespoon gelatin
½ teaspoon baking powder
¼ teaspoon salt
⅓ cup dark chocolate chips (55% cocoa)

1. Preheat the oven to 350°F. Grease an 8 x 8-inch baking pan with nonstick cooking spray.

2. In a large bowl, whisk together the butter, sweetener, eggs, and vanilla. Add the almond flour, cocoa powder, gelatin, baking powder, and salt and whisk until well combined. Stir in ¼ cup water to thin the batter. Stir in the chocolate chips.

3. Spread the batter in the prepared baking pan. Bake for 15 minutes, until the edges are set.

4. Remove and let cool completely in the pan.

5. Serve and enjoy!

Churro Mug Cake

Servings: 1

1 large egg
2 tablespoons butter
2 tablespoons almond flour
1 tablespoon Cruise Control–friendly sweetener
7 drops liquid stevia
½ teaspoon baking powder
¼ teaspoon cinnamon, plus more for serving
¼ teaspoon nutmeg
¼ teaspoon pure vanilla extract
Whipped cream (optional)

1. Mix together the egg, butter, almond flour, sweetener, liquid stevia, baking powder, cinnamon, nutmeg, and vanilla in a microwavable mug.

2. Microwave on high for 1 minute.

3. Turn the mug upside down on a plate and remove the cake. Top with whipped cream, if using, and a dash of cinnamon.

4. Serve and enjoy!

CHAPTER 7

The Exercise Effect

Exercise is the most potent yet
underutilized medicine.
—BILL PHILLIPS

So far we've almost exclusively talked about timing and food quality. Now we're going to turn our attention to movement, whether that amounts to an actual workout for you, or just getting off your couch and walking every day. Any amount of movement is beneficial for your health! But the kind of exercise that gets your heart thumping or that aims to build muscle is always a bonus—it'll boost your mood, increase your cognitive abilities, fight disease, decrease back and body pain, and lower heart disease risk. Exercise plus Cruise Control? Even better!

Like most people, you probably believe that you need to do structured, intense, and *long* workouts at the gym, in a class, or with focused running, spinning, or stair climbing, and so on. Because of many failed attempts at getting fit, maybe you gave up a long time ago. Perhaps you think it's too late, you've let things go for too long, you're too old, too fat, or that you were gifted frumpy, dumpy genes that make you powerless over getting the body of your dreams. None of these things are true. I promise. Because get this:

I'm about to make some big promises based on a workout that uses just two moves a day, and will only take you eight minutes to complete! If that doesn't sound crazy, how about this? With this workout, you can lose up to two pounds of fat each and every week in the time it takes to change the sheets on your bed.

What makes this workout uniquely effective is that you will have already primed your body to be a fat-burning machine with the way you are eating and thinking on Cruise Control. When you pair this automated lifestyle with easy exercises at the right time of day, you can have an eight-minute fitness routine that will yield big fitness results.

Now, if the idea of an eight-minute workout sounds familiar, you might be remembering my 2001 book called *8 Minutes in the Morning*. It was an instant bestseller, and one of the shortest, most efficient, and powerful weight-loss programs ever created, based on a compilation of science. It sold millions of copies around the globe. Why? Because no matter how busy you are, or how out of shape you are, or how much you travel for work, or how much your kids keep you up at night, or whatever you've been telling yourself that keeps you from exercising—you can find eight minutes a day to exercise! Pairing the fundamentals of my time-tested eight-minute moves with the belly fat burning machine you'll become on the Cruise Control Diet is the perfect combination!

LEARNING HOW TO EXERCISE FROM ANIMALS

There's something we can learn about exercise from animals. The next time you're playing outside with your dog, or when you watch an animal show on TV, or perhaps when you watch a video clip of kittens playing, I want you to notice how these animals move. Specifically, I want you to tell me when you see an animal jogging. That's right, jogging. You've never seen an animal jog, have you? You've seen a cheetah zooming after a gazelle, or a horse trotting, or your dog going for walks—but one thing you never see is an animal just jogging along for an hour a day or so. The reason is simple: At our most primal level, none of us—not animals and not humans—were designed for extended periods of low-intensity movement. Your body was made to either walk from point A to point B,

CATHY **SISNEROS**

AGE: 54 | WEIGHT LOST: 21 POUNDS

What everyone needs to know: You can stabilize your blood sugar and eliminate arthritis pain. I was thrilled to lose weight on Cruise Control, but I was even more excited when I got my new blood glucose meter and discovered that my blood sugar levels are now testing normal! I've been diabetic for many years and have always mostly controlled it with medications. This last spring my blood sugar really went out of control, and I didn't know what to do. Then I heard about Cruise Control and decided to give it a try. I'd heard that intermittent fasting could help with type 2 diabetes. But fasting for sixteen hours? No thanks. The Cruise Control loophole, fasting with fat during the Burn Zone, saved me. It makes "fasting" a breeze. I also was diagnosed with severe arthritis in my right knee and had been taking Naproxen for the pain on a regular basis. After Cruising for a few weeks I noticed that I no longer needed the medication, and last week I told my doctor I didn't need it anymore.

or to all-out sprint as fast as you can to get what you need (as in tracking down and hunting wildebeests or antelopes).

MOVEMENT IS MEDICINE FOR YOUR MIND

Have you ever noticed how you feel after an unusually active day? Maybe it was a day at the beach playing volleyball, or a family hike or bike ride, or perhaps you just got caught up last Sunday doing yard work—and while you might be tired and sore, I'll bet that you also have that good kind of tired feeling that comes from those extra active days. You feel calm, settled, serene, energized, and happy. It's no illusion. Exercise is as powerful as medicine in its effects on mood and physical health, according to a wealth of scientific research. Let's take a look.

A Better Mood: Physical activity stimulates the release of all sorts of feel-good chemicals—endorphins—in your brain. Which means it's really not a stretch to say that exercise is a mood enhancer. Or, as bestselling author Bill Phillips wrote in *Body for Life,* "Food is the most widely abused anti-anxiety drug in America, and exercise is the most potent and underutilized antidepressant." It's so true. In one Cochrane review, researchers analyzed twenty-three exercise and depression studies and concluded that exercise had a "large clinical impact" on depression. Another study, published in the *Archives of Internal Medicine,* found that exercise was as effective as the antidepressant Zoloft for those suffering from major depression.

Stress Relief: Regular participation in physical activity is empowering and confidence building. Research has also found that some team sports—racquetball, soccer, tennis, and even kickboxing and aerobics—build a team or herd mentality. And being part of a team reduces anxiety and relieves stress. In one study, published in the *American Journal of Psychiatry,* researchers chemically induced anxiety in two groups of adults: those who suffered from anxiety disorders and those who had just finished exercising for thirty minutes. Both groups got the same anxiety-producing chemical. While I wonder how this study got past the ethics committee, the authors found that the adults who exercised were less likely to have a panic response to the anxiety injection than those who were sedentary.

Enhanced Memory: Got brain fog? Get moving, say University of British Columbia researchers. In a study published in the *British Journal of Sports Medicine,* researchers found that people who engage in regular heart-pumping, sweat-producing exercise have a larger hippocampus (the area in your brain involved in memory and thinking) than those who don't exercise.

A Natural High: You've heard of the "runner's high," but many people regularly report that they feel a natural sense of euphoria after any sort of exercise. I see this with my clients all the time. They come in wound up, stressed out, agitated, and irritable, and they leave feeling great! In the past, research has pointed to the release of endorphins that trigger a response similar to opioid drugs. Recently, researchers in Germany discovered a different connection: the same area in the brain that is triggered to induce a high by the THC in marijuana also seems to be activated by exercise.

SHORT BURSTS OF EXERCISE BOOST YOUR BURN BETTER

Many health experts recommend that you get an hour of moderate-level exercise or more a day. But did you know that this recommendation is in regards to maintaining your weight and improving your health—but it won't burn off fat? There is actually no research that backs up using this type of exercise specifically for weight loss. Wait. What? You read correctly. I've been a trainer for twenty years, and I'm telling you something that the American College of Sports Medicine, the American Council on Exercise, and thousands of other fitness experts around the world have long known: you will not burn fat—and certainly not belly fat—with sixty minutes of moderate-intensity exercise. Not even if you do it seven days a week.

Now, I'm not saying that exercising for an hour a day is terrible. I highly recommend movement all throughout the day, but it doesn't have to be sweat-drenched at the gym. Any time you move, your health will benefit from it. But your belly fat? It's persistent, and it needs something special. You are already doing that "something special" by following the Cruise Control Diet. Following a steady Boost and Burn Zone each day gives you the intermittent fasting you need to turn on your body's fat-burning engine. My eight-minute workout provides another boost to your already revved fat-burning engine. It's this boost that ramps up the belly burning.

CATECHOLAMINES: BOOSTING YOUR BURN

Catecholamines are a group of hormones and neurotransmitters that your body pumps out in response to stress—and they prompt your body to boost fat burning. How? Adrenaline.

Catecholamines are typically activated when your fight-or-flight reaction is triggered. You know: you perceive a threat or danger, adrenaline is released, your heart speeds up, digestion slows, blood is sent to your major muscle groups, yada yada . . . it gives your body a burst of energy, so you are ready to do battle or to skedaddle—fast.

Catecholamines are also activated and release adrenaline in response to one type of exercise: high-intensity interval training (HIIT). HIIT is a method of exercise that requires you to alternate intervals of all-out effort (like sprinting at your fastest) for a short amount of time with moderate-intensity exercise (a brisk walk). According to a study published in the *Journal of Obesity* by researchers from the University of South Wales in Australia, HIIT resulted in a greater fat loss (with the majority coming from belly fat) when compared to steady-state exercise. The study followed women who did these training sessions just three times a week. If that's not interesting enough, consider this: researchers who have looked at elite tennis players find that they burn belly fat before any other place in the body. You'd think that these athletes would be burning off the fat in their arms or legs. The thinking is that tennis is an entire game of HIIT bursts, and so it is better at burning the hardest, most unbudgeable fat—what lives around your middle.

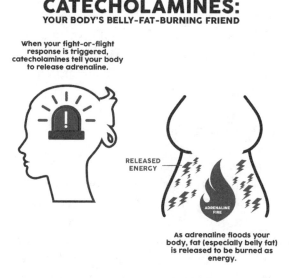

CATECHOLAMINES:
YOUR BODY'S BELLY-FAT-BURNING FRIEND

When your fight-or-flight response is triggered, catecholamines tell your body to release adrenaline.

RELEASED ENERGY

ADRENALINE FIRE

As adrenaline floods your body, fat (especially belly fat) is released to be burned as energy.

What do you think the eight minutes of exercise I prescribe are? Yes—HIIT exercises!

As I've said, moderate cardio exercise (if any), such as walking, jogging, riding a bike, and so on, is great for mood boosting and improving the health of your lungs, heart, and circulation, and for increasing your life span, but it won't spot-burn belly fat. Even if you go to the gym for an intense spin class or to lift weights for an hour (also great for burning calories and getting strong, respectively), you won't flatten your belly. That pooch just sticks around.

Instead of logging hours at the gym, the Cruise Control Workout uses alternate periods of short, intense anaerobic exercise with less-intense recovery periods. I promise this isn't complicated, only two moves that work together to boost your mood, increase your life span, and condition all the muscles in your body—yep, to effectively torch belly fat.

EXERCISE BOOSTS THE CRUISE CONTROL FAT-BURNING LIFESTYLE

First, let me reiterate: you will already be burning body and belly fat by eating and "fasting with fat" the Cruise Control way. Your exercise routine will boost your mood and increase your life span, and *as a bonus*, it will amplify the fat burning that is already happening thanks to Boosting and Burning each day.

Remember, animals move in short, explosive bursts of energy to get what they need and you need to, too. To set off that catecholamine, you need small, short bursts of energy. These are exact principles around which I designed the Cruise Control Workout.

When to Move for Maximum Fat Burning

As a practical matter, I recommend exercising near the end of your Burn Zone (in the morning). This is when your body starts burning glycogen, the limited sugar stored in the liver. Since there is extra demand for energy during exercise, this will make your glycogen run out faster. That's a good thing because then your body can turn to burning fat. This doesn't happen to people who wake up and immediately eat. Remember, most Americans spike blood sugar for fifteen or more hours a day—not you! You are going to run out of glycogen much faster because you've been in the Burn Zone for close to sixteen hours. Your body will have already used some of the limited glycogen available in your liver while you were sleeping. Less glycogen in the Burn Zone means a fast lane to fat burning, especially when you pair the morning Burn Zone with the Cruise Control Workout.

You've heard of athletes who "hit the wall"? This usually happens in a body that is still primarily burning sugar, not fat. In this case, the body taps out because the glycogen in the liver is limited, but your body hasn't adapted to using fat for energy—that's what causes the "hit the wall" effect. That won't happen on Cruise Control because following the Boost and Burn Zones will quickly make your body efficient at burning fat. Your fat-burning ability is even more enhanced at the end of your Burn Zone.

All this is not to say that you won't get any benefit if you need to train midday, in the afternoon, or in the evening. The Boost and Burn Zones will still keep you fat-burning at all times of the day so your body will be energized whenever you decide to do your workout. That said, you'll be most highly primed to burn fat in the morning because you will have been in a fasted state the longest at this time.

By exercising before your first meal of the day, you hasten the burning of the limited sugar (glycogen) stored in your liver, which means that your body can get to burning fat for energy faster. Now, does it make sense to exercise for longer than these eight-minute moves or at other times of the day? Sure, if you want. Including an extra hour of moderate movement such as walking, biking, elliptical, Stairmaster training, or a workout class will give your health and happiness a boost. Need to do your workouts later in the day? No problem. You'll still see benefits and fat burning. I'm just letting you know when you'll get the *most* massive transformation: in the morning, for eight minutes, and two moves.

Muscle Burns Fat: Muscle cells are better at taking up glucose when you have fasted for a period of time, and that's what you'll be doing in your Burn Zone. Your insulin sensitivity increases within cells, and so does the uptake of amino acids. That means better energy balance and production. Then you exercise, which puts more immediate stress on the muscle cells. The cells are highly primed to pick up energy and amino acids and to grow and rebuild muscle proteins.

Muscle Makes You Lean and Sleek: Talk of building muscle scares some of my female clients. They picture themselves getting big and bulky, but that's not how Cruise Control works. Muscle burns more calories and takes up less than half the space fat does—so you look sleek and slim, not like the Incredible Hulk when he's having a bad day.

Burning Melts Fat Faster: You are going to see more fat loss when you exercise in your Burn Zone than at any other time of the day. As you may have read in earlier chapters, much of the caloric value of the food you eat is stored in the liver as glycogen (remember, it's limited). In the Burn Zone, you quickly use up that glycogen and start burning fat. Side note: this will happen whether you exercise or not. Just going about your day will eventually burn off your glycogen stores and your body will begin tapping into the fat, but you can ramp this up with just a little moving at any time of the day, but especially in the morning.

Travel with Cruise Control

My passion is coming up with simple solutions to complex problems, so the entire Cruise Control method is designed to travel with you anywhere you go, and my scientifically backed workout is no exception. You can do it wherever you happen to go, and you'll take the body and belly fat burning with you.

While my Cruise Control is effortless to do anywhere, if you want to mix it up or if you have a particular method of working out that you're partial to, there's no need to give it up. You can get the same results by simply applying the same interval training technique behind my workout to a whole host of exercises. So please, continue to spin, run, walk, lift weights, Zumba, and Jazzercise; just weave in some high-intensity moves with more moderate ones, and you're good to go. Cruise Control is made to work with you as you travel the long road of a healthy and happy life.

MY TECH GUARDIAN TO BETTER HEALTH

I am always searching for a smarter way to stay motivated with fitness. For me there are two things I tell all my celebrity clients that are essential to today's modern world. The first is to have the right technology and the second is to have the right support system and environment.

Technology has been a big help, and if you follow me on social media you might be able to spot that I am always wearing a fitness tracker on my wrist. My top pick is the Apple Watch, specifically the 4 Series. I like the size of the screen (bigger than past generations) and the fact that it's got a really thin profile—I sometimes even forget it's there! The secret weapon on this watch is the Activity App; it's critical in tracking three vital pieces of information. It has an electrocardiogram (ECG) monitor that measures the electrical activity of your heart, as well as data on irregular heart rhythms. It'll even let you know if you may be experiencing dangerous irregularities. The second thing it tracks is when you move by showing you how many active calories you've burned throughout the day. Finally, it tracks your exercise by monitoring any brisk activity you've done throughout the day, such as the HIIT workouts in this book. With an emphasis on Stand, Move, and Exercise, you will constantly be reminded to sit less (such as when you're relaxing at the pool), move more (such as by taking a hike), and do some brisk activity (such as HIIT)!

The gym is my other surefire source of motivation. Variety is essential to sustaining your interest—no matter how much you love running, I guarantee there will be a day when you just don't feel like it, and when you don't see other options around you, that's when it's easy to quit moving. Research also shows that variety is essential for your body to get stronger and for your brain to get smarter. When you've mastered a movement, your muscle fibers and your neural networks are no longer challenged—and that's when changes to your body slow down (athletes call it plateauing). You might not feel as energized and serene, and you might even feel bored or "burned out." That's why 24 Hour Fitness is one of my favorite gym chains, offering not only the strength and cardio equipment, studio and workout spaces, but also a huge variety of classes that come with membership, as well as a free app to personalize and use when you're at the gym and when you're not. I love partnering with them as they have a comprehensive understanding that fitness is a lifestyle and that mindset, workouts, nutrition, and recovery combine together for results. Most important to me, though, is the sense of community that comes with the familiar faces in your class, on the workout floor or at the front desk. It won't take long for you to look forward to a friendly smile or a coffee after a good sweat session, and sometimes that's all you really need to get going. See Resources in Appendix B for more information.

If that all sounds great to you but you're not sure where to start, many gyms offer coaching, and at 24 Hour Fitness you'll even get a custom workout plan, designed by a professional trainer, to get you started. Having trouble getting through the door? What always works is taking a small step that easily becomes habit: Lay out your gym clothes or pack your bag the night before and put it by the door. If you prefer to work out in the morning, it's not hard to roll out of bed and into comfy gym clothes; if you like to take a lunch break outside the office, that gym bag by your desk is pretty hard to ignore. Once you've got those shoes on, it's hard not to take the next step—you might as well go!

CHAPTER 8

Your Cruise Control Workout

The only way you can hurt your
body is if you don't use it.
—JACK LALANNE

So, without further ado, here is the workout you've been waiting for! At eight minutes a day, five times a week, we're talking about just forty minutes per week, which is all you need to activate the powerful fat-mobilizing hormones and neurotransmitters that will burn off your belly fat in a way that's far more effective than long, intense exercise sessions. All it takes is your commitment and participation.

I always say that most weight-loss programs fail because they take so much time or are so restrictive that even if you're trying your best, it's difficult to make it work unless you take an actual break from real life (like the type of thing you see on reality TV). Since most of us don't have that luxury, I designed these moves to help you succeed no matter how jam-packed your schedule or your life—I created this to succeed for you no matter what!

How it works is simple. You'll warm up for a few minutes. You will alternate a one-minute high-intensity move with a one-minute low-intensity move for a total of eight minutes. You'll cool down for a few minutes and then get on with your day. Finito. It's time to take action!

Note: While this exercise portion of Cruise Control *is* optional, I do highly recommend it (it's eight minutes). That said, if you decide not to use the exercises, *do commit to moving* your body every single day.

WHAT YOU'LL NEED

- Good fitness shoes
- A room with space to move
- Your favorite music

THE BREAKDOWN

High-Intensity Moves: Introducing the Most Intense Sixty Seconds of Your Day

To temporarily stress your body so it can burn fat, especially in an eight-minute workout, your aim is to do these moves at an intensity of 80 to 95 percent of your total energy output (see the chart "How to Measure Your Intensity" page 210), but just for that one minute. You want heart rate pumping fast and your muscles fatigued. You'll be engaging all of your large muscle groups and many smaller ones as well, to mimic how our ancestors moved while on the hunt. This is what will torch the fat that is currently padding your body.

When you are moving at this intensity, you shouldn't be able to talk, and by the end of the last move (at the end of eight minutes), you'll be sweating like a, well, you'll be sweating profusely. While you want to move quickly, that doesn't mean that you are loosely flopping your arms and legs about. Make these moves rapid, with control and proper form. You want to finish each of these one-minute moves feeling like you couldn't do another second more. Aim to be at an 8- or 9-level intensity during the high-intensity movement.

Low-Intensity Moves: The Importance of Active Recovery

Continuing to move between high-intensity exercises speeds up the removal of lactic acid and helps lower bloodstream acidity that can make muscles burn and that slows you down. A simpler way to look at it: keeping your body moving gives you the energy you need to ramp back up for the next high-intensity interval. Each one-minute active-recovery move improves your blood circulation and muscle recovery and keeps your stress levels low, and you feeling happy. You want to do these exercises in a controlled manner, concentrating on contracting the muscles in each targeted move. Your one-minute recovery move will continue to condition and strengthen to build lean muscle. Aim to be at a 6- to 7-level intensity during active recovery.

HOW TO MEASURE YOUR INTENSITY

0 TO 1:	No Intensity. You might be asleep.
2 TO 3:	Easy intensity. You begin at 10 percent intensity and move up to 50 percent intensity. You are just starting your warm-up.
4 TO 5:	Semi-easy intensity. You are at 60 to 70 percent intensity. Your breathing and heart rate are picking up, and your body feels warmer. You can still easily carry on a conversation.
6 TO 7:	Low to moderate intensity: You are at 70 to 80 percent intensity. It's getting a little harder to talk, and you are sweating, but you aren't yet gasping for air.
8 TO 9:	High intensity: This is where you reach your 85 to 90 percent intensity. Now you're breathing hard, and you are sweating like a beast. You can only say a short word or two if you must, and you'd rather not. You can't keep this up for much longer.
10	All-out uber-high intensity: 95 to 100 percent intensity. You can't speak, your muscles are burning, and there's a puddle of sweat between your feet. You can't do this for more than forty seconds.

Modifications: It's Your Workout! If you find a move too difficult or too easy, modify it. You are in the driver's seat, so you decide. The goal is for you to be able to tap into the intensity to keep your body burning fat. Remember that even if you start out with modifications, later you'll be able to add extra minutes to your workout.

Make It Easier: Some of the exercises are compound exercises that involve numerous movements or require explosive actions. If an activity feels too complicated or difficult, take it down a notch by grabbing a chair for support or decreasing the intensity a bit. You can also cut down the sixty seconds to thirty seconds if you need a gradual approach. You'll still see amazing results from all the other components of Cruise Control. You'll get stronger as the weeks move forward, and you'll soon be mastering all the moves.

Make It Harder: If you want a harder workout, or if you don't feel like you're reaching the recommended 85 to 90 percent intensity, check your pace and be sure that you're pushing yourself during both high- and low-intensity moves. Still too easy? Ramp it up! Add a jump, hop, or jog; make your arms move more explosively and powerfully; or add extra focus to engaging the muscles targeted in the exercise (always with control and good form). As you move through the twenty-eight-day program, if you still don't feel like you're hitting the right speed (you're no longer breaking a sweat or feeling the burn in your muscles), you can repeat the workout for a total of sixteen minutes. The stronger you get, the more times you'll be able to Cruise through the eight-minute drill at a higher intensity than when you started. You can do as many rounds as you want—sixteen, twenty-four, thirty-two, or forty minutes—it's up to you! You can also add weights or kettlebells to the moves where it makes sense. Hint: I love the kettlebells you can get from Kettlebell Kings because they have a softer coating on the outside (for more information, see Resources, page 313). Remember, if the workout starts to feel easier, it's a sign that you're getting fitter, leaner, and stronger.

Warming Up and Cooling Down: Before and after every workout, take a few minutes to move your body around to get it ready for your workout and to transition back down when you are done. Walk in place, jog gently, circle your arms, lift and lower your shoulders, lift and lower your knees, or dance around—any sort of movement will do.

YOUR FOUR-WEEK PLAN

Remember, each workout consists of four cycles of two exercises for eight minutes:

WARM UP	Low intensity to moderate intensity	2 to 3 minutes
CYCLE 1	Move 1: High Intensity	60 seconds
	Move 2: Moderate Intensity	60 seconds
CYCLE 2	Move 1: High Intensity	60 seconds
	Move 2: Moderate Intensity	60 seconds
CYCLE 3	Move 1: High Intensity	60 seconds
	Move 2: Moderate Intensity	60 seconds
CYCLE 4	Move 1: High Intensity	60 seconds
	Move 2: Moderate Intensity	60 seconds
COOL DOWN	Low intensity to moderate intensity	2 to 3 minutes

Day One: Arms & Abs

EXERCISE 1: ALTERNATING OVERHEAD PRESS

Description: Stand with your feet about hip-width apart, knees slightly bent. Lift your arms overhead, so both arms are straight and your hands are in fists facing each other. Bend your right arm to bring your fist down to shoulder height; your elbow is pointing down toward the floor. Punch your right arm back up, and as you do, bring your left arm down, so your fist is at shoulder height, elbow pointing down. Continue alternating arms, punching upward for 60 seconds. Go to Exercise 2.

IMAGE SEQUENCE

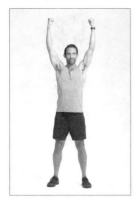 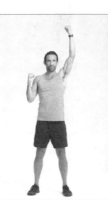 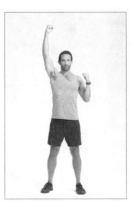

| START | MIDDLE | FINISH |

EXERCISE 2: OVERHEAD MARCH

Description: Stand with your feet about hip-width apart and hold both arms straight overhead as you march in place, bringing alternating knees up toward your chest for 60 seconds. Repeat Alternating Overhead Press.

IMAGE SEQUENCE

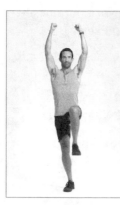 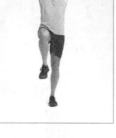 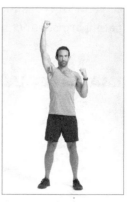

START   **MIDDLE**   **FINISH**

Day Two: Butt & Legs

EXERCISE 1: ALTERNATING GATE SQUATS

Description: Stand with your feet shoulder-width apart, knees slightly bent. Your arms are bent, elbows down, and hands in loose fists on either side of your chin. Take a wide step to your right side and squat down as far as you comfortably can (make sure your knees stay behind your toes). Push back into your heels and stand back up, bringing your right foot back to the starting stance. Immediately step out to your left and squat down in the same manner. Continue alternating sides for 60 seconds. Proceed to Exercise 2.

IMAGE SEQUENCE

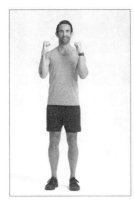 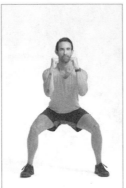 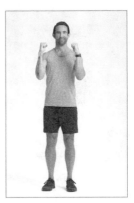

START   **MIDDLE**   **FINISH**

EXERCISE 2: SKATER GLUTE PULSE

Description: Stand with your feet hip-width apart and arms overhead, your fingertips toward the ceiling. Take a step forward with your left foot and bend slightly forward from your hips; your front leg is slightly bent and your back leg is straight. From here, lift your right foot, supporting yourself on your left leg. Press your right heel up and contract your glute (butt). Continue lifting and lowering for 30 seconds. Stand back up, and repeat on the other side, for 30 seconds. Repeat Alternating Gate Squats.

IMAGE SEQUENCE

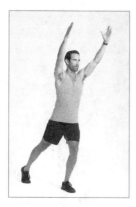

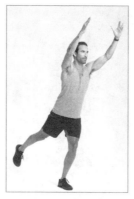

START   FINISH

Day Three: Chest & Back

EXERCISE 1: STANDING PUSH-UPS WITH SHOULDER TAPS

Description: Stand with your arms straight out in front of you. As if you were doing an imaginary push-up, pull your arms back, bringing your shoulder blades together, then straighten your arms back out in front of you, and then immediately tap opposite shoulders with each hand and repeat from the start. Continue for 60 seconds. Proceed to Exercise 2.

IMAGE SEQUENCE

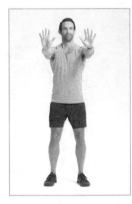

START

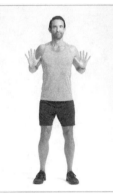

MIDDLE 1

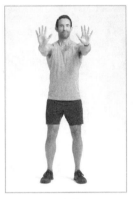

MIDDLE 2

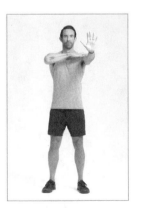

MIDDLE 3

FINISH

EXERCISE 2: YTW

Description: Stand with your feet a little wider than hip-width, and bend forward about 45 degrees from the hip. Lift and lower your arms straight up to form the letter Y with your body; hold for 5 seconds. Now bring your arms out to the side, palms up, to form the letter T, hold for 5 seconds, and then bend your arms so your elbows point toward the floor and your arms form the letter W and hold for 5 seconds. Continue cycling through each YTW for 60 seconds total. Repeat Exercise 1.

IMAGE SEQUENCE

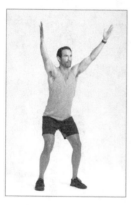
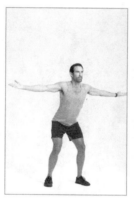
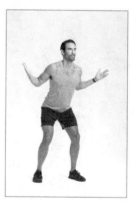

START   MIDDLE   FINISH

FOCUS ON FORM

When you get tired, and your muscles start burning, you may well be cursing every single rep you have left to do. And it's at that exact moment of fatigue that one critical element of your workout may start to suffer: form. Shoulders roll forward, knees dip where they're not supposed to. But remember this: Bad form can cause severe injuries. As the song goes, check yourself before you wreck yourself.

- Be sure to follow the exercise descriptions carefully.
- Invest in a $5 tall mirror (stores like Target have these—they're lightweight and don't even need to be mounted). Use it every time you work out. Or enlist a Cruiser and be each other's mirrors.
- While you should be moving as fast as you can to make sure you're reaching the right level of intensity, it's still more important to do fewer proper reps than more sloppy ones. As you get stronger and more accustomed to the moves, your pace will pick up. But don't learn to do these the wrong way from the get-go.
- If you absolutely must rest to regain proper form, do it. As the weeks fly by, you'll be able to skip the rest periods.

Day Four: Core

EXERCISE 1: STIR THE POT

Description: Stand tall, feet hip-width apart, with your core engaged. Make a fist with your right hand, and cover it with your left. Now, as if you are stirring a ginormous pot of stew, start making large circles with your arms, keeping your hands together. After a few rotations in one direction, switch your hands, right over left fist, and "stir" the pot the other direction. Continue alternating for 60 seconds. Proceed to Exercise 2.

IMAGE SEQUENCE

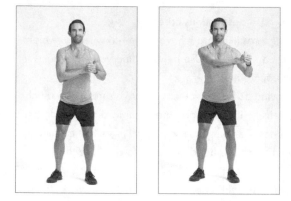

START   **MIDDLE 1**

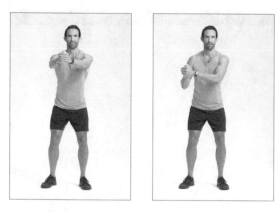

MIDDLE 2   **FINISH**

EXERCISE 2: ALTERNATING PRISONER TWIST MARCH

Description: Stand tall with your feet hip-width apart, hands behind your head, and elbows out of sight to either side. Keeping your core muscles tight, rotate your shoulders to the left as you lift your left knee up toward the sky. Repeat with the other side, rotating in the other direction. Continue alternating sides for 60 seconds. If you need to pause between sides, that's okay. Just get back to moving as soon as you feel able. Repeat Exercise 1.

IMAGE SEQUENCE

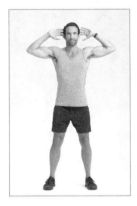 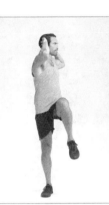 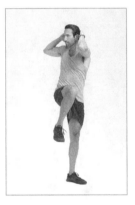

| START | MIDDLE | FINISH |

Complete exercises, alternating 1 and 2 for four rounds, or for a total of eight minutes.

Day Five: Total Body

EXERCISE 1: SQUAT PLUS TOE PRESS

Description: Stand with feet a little wider than hip-width apart. Bend your knees and sit back as far as you comfortably can. Press into your heels and as you stand back up, press up onto the balls of your feet. Lower back onto your heels with control, and continue to repeat the move for 60 seconds. Proceed to Exercise 2.

IMAGE SEQUENCE

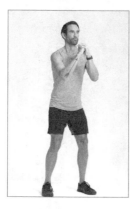

START

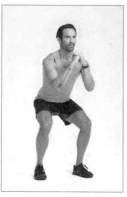

MIDDLE 1

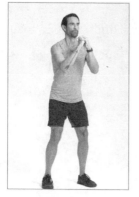

MIDDLE 2

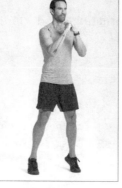

FINISH

EXERCISE 2: ALTERNATING THIGH MARCH

Description: Stand tall with your feet under your hips, upper arms at your side, elbows bent at 90 degrees, palms facing the floor. Bend your leg forward to bring one knee up to tap the palm on the same side. Lower your leg and repeat with the other side. Continue alternating sides for 60 seconds. Repeat Exercise 1.

IMAGE SEQUENCE

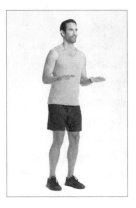
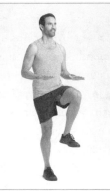
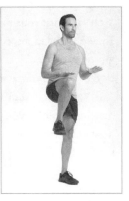

| START | MIDDLE | FINISH |

Complete exercises, alternating 1 and 2 for four rounds, or for a total of eight minutes.

HOW DO I "ENGAGE" MY CORE?

If you read fitness articles or books, exercises often come with the recommendation to "engage" your core or your muscles. But when I meet with clients, many of them don't know what this means or how to do it. It isn't difficult, and it's super important to building sleek, lean muscle, burning fat, and getting your intensity where it needs to go. Here are a few tips.

It's not just your belly: The "core" includes your back, butt, and stomach. They are called the core because they work as a team to keep your head on top of your shoulders and support your neck, spine, and pelvis to give you a stable center from which you can operate your head, arms, and legs.

It's different from sucking in your tummy: Imagine you are about to be punched right in your stomach. What would you do? You instinctively know how to clench and brace the muscles in your core if you visualize being hit in the middle. This is engaging your core, but there's another piece to it. While you want to brace your core, you don't want to do it with your tummy pooching out. So check that your tummy is pulled in as you brace your core.

Maintain good posture at all times: Whether you are standing, sitting, or lying on your back, you still want to keep a natural curve in your spine, keep your head and neck in line with your torso (not tilted forward or back), and keep from slouching.

Engage other muscles: You can use the same "you are about to be punched" visualization for other parts of your body. Try it now. Visualize that someone is going to hit you in your upper arm. See how you automatically tighten up your arm muscles? You can do this with any part of your body.

Don't flop: To always have a fantastic workout, use control. You want to move quickly in the high-intensity moves, but you always want to maintain good form and control. If you just fling your arms and legs about, you won't get the fat-burning, muscle-building workout results. Ditto on moderate-intensity. Always use good form and control.

END-OF-WEEK MANDATORY RECOVERY TREATS

At the end of your week of workouts, be sure to reward yourself to a recovery treat, such as getting a massage or having a relaxing spa treatment. One thing I recently tried that I love was cryotherapy, which is a cooling therapy that's done in a really fast, really intense way that takes only three minutes. You get really cold, but you also relieve all your aches and pains because it provides a fast, full-body anti-inflammation treatment. It's pretty awesome, definitely faster than a pain reliever. You can find places that will give you a cryotherapy facial, which can be a good introduction to the whole cold-therapy revolution. However, I really like the full-body treatment I got from Cryo Science. I felt extremely energized after my three minutes, and I find that this therapy works extremely well for my clients who have joint pain or arthritis. For more information, see Resources, page 316.

Rest Day and Alternative Activities

You may already be well on your way to seeing results, especially if you've put in a week or two of sticking with the Cruise Control Workout and eating suggestions. You may want to do more, and if so, I say, go right ahead! Adding in extra cycles of the workout is great because the more time you spend doing high-intensity interval training (HIIT), the more fat you'll burn. That said, it's important to focus on the quality of your moves, not just quantity. That means if you keep pushing past the point that you can maintain good form with the exercises, it's a clue to wrap it up.

Take a rest day when you need it, but a "rest" day doesn't mean sitting on the sofa bingeing on Netflix all day. Your rest days can be spent any way you like, but I encourage you to consider doing something enjoyable that involves moving your body. This might be some intimate time rolling around in the hay with your loved one, heading out for a bike ride or a stroll with your family or a friend, gardening, or doing other active chores around the house. Use your rest days to allow your body to keep your circulation going at a low to moderate intensity so your body can repair and rejuvenate. Doing this will prepare you to have loads of energy for your next eight-minute workout.

REJUVENATE YOUR RECOVERY

Everyone always asks me about the best way to recover after a workout. It's obviously important to hydrate and fuel yourself after exercise, but to take your recovery to the next level, some innovative therapies have caught my eye recently. One of these is to use natural light therapy that counters the fatigue-causing and sleep-disrupting lights and screens that we are typically exposed to during the majority of our waking hours. I really like the natural light therapy available from a company called Joovv. Here's why. After a good workout, your cells are depleted, and your body starts working overtime to produce more cellular energy. Exposing your cells to natural red and near-infrared light from a Joovv light machine stimulates your cells to recharge your mitochondria, which kick-starts the recovery process. I've noticed that it helps with strained muscles and joint mobility. I feel less stiff and sore after I have a session of red light therapy. After I fractured my ankle, my doctor suggested light therapy to help boost the collagen for faster healing and to help relieve my pain from the break. I was amazed at how fast I recovered and was able to get back to training clients. I haven't stopped using light therapy since. Red light therapy is a paradigm shift in the world of training and recovery, and it's backed by tons of clinical research. It builds my clients' muscle strength so they can perform at their peak, and the energy boost makes workouts more effective and efficient. Find more information in the Resources, page 315.

There are literally a ton of activities you can do on your rest days. Here are a few ideas.

- **Go for a Walk:** This is about the easiest thing you could ever do and is right in line with how your body is meant to move. Remember how animals walk or run, they don't jog? Taking a walk is a great way to help your body recover, and it provides some great benefits as well. Studies find that walking improves memory in people over age fifty. It's an easy, natural movement that doesn't really engage your brain intensely, which means you have the mindful space to reflect on your life circumstances, you can problem-solve, or you can even meditate. Walks are also a great activity to share with someone else. These should be at a leisurely pace that lets you enjoy chatting, or, as I like to call it, "time to solve the problems of the world."

- **Ride a Bike:** A truly joyful ride. No matter your age or fitness level, you can enjoy the scenery and feeling the wind on your face just like when you were a kid. Another benefit of pedaling: it can help keep you feeling happy! In a survey conducted by Portland State University, respondents who biked to work reported the highest levels of well-being.

- **Try a Yoga Class:** One of my clients' favorite "rest" day activities is yoga, often because it provides luxurious stretches for hardworking muscles. While their flexibility improves, so does strength as yoga incorporates movements like the plank, which not only tones muscles but helps you become stronger for your workout. Other yoga benefits are wonderful, too, like helping you get a better night's sleep! A study reported in *Medical Science Monitor* found that patients with sleep problems reported an improved quality of their sleep on days when they did yoga and meditation. It also releases feel-good chemicals in your brain. Scientists at Boston University School of Medicine and McLean Hospital were able to see that people who did yoga for thirty minutes had a 27 percent increase of gamma-aminobutyric acid (GABA) in their brains. This feel-good chemical helps regulate nerve activity—it's reduced in people with mood and anxiety disorders, so the goal is to have more if you want to feel happier and more relaxed.

- **Take a Hike:** Most of us live within driving distance of some beautiful nature. Get up close and personal with all of Mother Nature's splendor by taking a hike. It's one of my favorite ways to leave behind the hustle, bustle, and fast pace of everyday life. Make sure to take along your smartphone, not just to snap photos, but to make the most out of some helpful hiking apps, like AllTrails, a free GPS tracker that uploads real-time information on your location and condition. Bring a friend along, too, especially if you're heading somewhere without a lot of foot traffic.

- **Lift Weights:** Although strength-training moves are incorporated in my workout, they focus on using your own body as your barbell, so to speak. If you enjoy lifting weights—or want to give it a try—now's a great time to start. When Penn State researchers put dieters into three groups—no exercise, aerobic exercise only, or aerobic exercise and weight training—they all lost around twenty-one pounds. But those who worked out with weights lost six more pounds of fat than the non-lifting participants. That's because lifting weights helped them to build and retain muscle. Other research shows that dieters who don't lift weights or participate in resistance training lose 25 percent of their weight from muscle instead of fat. Something else to think about: as we age, bone mass decreases, which increases your likelihood of suffering a fracture. But research has found that sixteen weeks of resistance training increased hip bone density and elevated blood levels of osteocalcin—a marker of bone growth—by 19 percent. While you're getting resistance training through Cruise Control moves, this is a different way to get more—and one you can do on "rest" days.

- **Move with Something New:** On rest days it's important to engage your entire body with some sort of movement, whether that be passive or active recovery. Switch things up and try out a piece of exercise equipment like an elliptical or punching bag. Or jump around with a trampoline or jump rope to work both your upper and lower body. A gym like 24 Hour Fitness is my top pick for variety when I'm not sure what I'd like to try. Besides a wide variety of equipment, classes, training spaces, basketball courts and swimming pools, there are knowledgeable and helpful group fitness instructors and personal trainers who are available to suggest options based on your workout preferences and goals, and focused on ones that you might enjoy and that will add variety to your routine—and, of course, to show you how to use a piece of equipment that caught your eye. **Vasper** is my favorite full-body exercise machine because it combines compression and cooling technology to reduce pain and deliver more oxygen to your muscles. I learned about this from my good friend and colleague Tony Robbins, and now I use this frequently on Sundays. I call it "My 21-Minute Miracle" and I always feel energized and rejuvenated after. See Resources in Appendix B for more information.

- **Sweat It Out in a Sauna:** I love saunas. I have a heating pad that I can use on my achy joints at home, but it doesn't give me the all-over relief I feel when my muscles are sore from an extra-intense workout. The only thing I've found for that is sitting in a sauna. It's a relaxing way to support your Cruise Control program. For more information, see "Saunas for Weight Loss," page 231.

- **Put on Your Dancing Shoes:** One of the best things that my Cruisers report is experiencing confidence that they never thought they'd feel. It's the feeling that comes with working hard and experiencing success! And that fabulous new feeling often makes it easier to try something you've always thought would be fun but were a little timid about actually doing. For a lot of people, that's dancing. Some have always wanted to try a popular dance class like Zumba. For others, it could be signing up for ballroom dance classes with their spouse. What a great way to get some social—or one-on-one—time and do it while moving your body. Besides being a fun activity on your "rest" days, I absolutely love this idea for date night—instead of going out to a heavy dinner. No significant other? No problem. Most ballroom dance schools offer options for singles, too—like group salsa classes.

- **Do Some Gardening:** Gardening is excellent moderate cardio exercise. I'm not talking about gently watering a few plants, mind you. However, if you pull weeds, dig a new planting area, mow the lawn, or rake the leaves, you can burn up to 300 calories in forty-five minutes, and you'll work out your arms, back, butt, and legs. You'll also give your arteries, heart, and lungs the type of exercise that keeps them flexible and healthy. Plus, you get the mood-boosting benefits of being in natural daylight.

- **Speed Clean:** Are you avoiding vacuuming up the pet hair and mopping the kitchen floor? You might be motivated to know that you can organize your chores in a way that won't only leave you with a sparkling clean house, but you'll get a great workout to boot. Here's how I do it. Get out all your cleaning equipment and products and put them in one central location. Plan to clean from top to bottom, not from room to room. For example, grab your rags and your wood and counter cleaners, and start with your kitchen counters and cabinets, stove, and other appliances. Then do your dining room, living room, and bedroom furniture dusting—don't forget the bathroom counters and the top of the toilet. Move briskly, no breaks. Now go back to the cleaners and equipment and switch to your sweeping and vacuuming. Do as much of the house as you can. Keep up the brisk pace. Then go back to your equipment, fill up your bucket, grab your mop, and go to it. My favorite way to end is throwing down two large rags on the wet floors and then stepping on them and shuffling around on them to dry the floors. It's great for a leg and core workout. You can burn up to 300 calories doing this speed-cleaning routine.

- **My 21-Minute Miracle:** Another way to take the power of cooling and put it into action for your recovery and performance is with an amazing piece of ingenuity called Vasper. While Vasper may look like a recumbent stationary bike, it is actually a cutting-edge technology that combines compression, cooling, and interval training to increase your body's production of strength and bone-building hormones. During a Vasper session, the compression cuffs on your arms and legs fill up with cold water and squeeze your limbs during a twenty-one-minute "ride" that involves short bursts of high intensity and then low-intensity recovery (same as the Cruise Control Workout). This stimulates body's production of the hormones that help you lose weight, and enhance performance and recovery. The cooling improves your performance by making your workout feel far easier than a traditional high-intensity workout, but you'll mimic the physiology of an intensive two hour session. Vasper is a powerful compliment to all other exercise and is the best substitute for exercise when you are pressed for time (see the Resources section, page 313, for more information).

SAUNAS FOR WEIGHT LOSS

I know it sounds suspicious, but there's actually some good research on using certain kinds of saunas to help lose weight and to support a healthy weight. In a 2009 study, Sunlighten infrared saunas were shown to help lower weight and waist circumference in just a three-month period. The common theme among subjects in the study was that infrared sauna use was similar to moderate exercise but "much more relaxing." So these saunas can be an effective support to weight loss and fat burning, especially if you are unable to do the Cruise Control Workout due to conditions such as osteoarthritis or cardiovascular or respiratory problems. In addition, according to information published in the *Journal of the American Medical Association,* infrared sauna weight-loss sessions were shown to burn up to 600 calories. The reason seems to be that these sauna sessions increase core temperatures, which causes your body to burn calories in the process of cooling itself. That's also why you sweat. I take a sauna daily to detoxify and recover. It's my favorite place to read and relax. See Resources, page 315, for more information.

FUEL YOUR WORKOUT

One thing I always do during and after an intense workout is make sure that I'm rehydrating and getting enough electrolytes. Your cells need electrolytes to stay stable and to carry electrical charges needed for nerve cells to communicate. When you do intense exercise, you can sweat out too many of your electrolytes, and many sports drinks that boast electrolytes also come with a bunch of sugar and other chemicals. I've found one that is totally natural that I love called LyteShow; ordering information is in the Resources section, page 311. It's a concentrate that you add to water, it adds a lemony tang, and it lasts for weeks. Plus, hydrating and lost electrolytes is the number one reason you can feel false hunger, so these drinks are important both pre- and post-workout. Also, I feel great after I have a drink of it. Here's a short list of other foods that will help fuel your body before and after your workout.

Pre-Workout

BURN ZONE

Apple cider vinegar diluted in water
Cruise Control Coffee
Fruit-infused water
Ginseng tea
Green tea
Matcha
Small glass of unsweetened milk
Water with Himalayan pink salt
Water with lemon

BOOST ZONE

Avocado
Cheese stick
FBOMBs (see Resources, page 303)
Handful of nuts
Hard-boiled egg
Jerky

Nut butter
Protein shake (see Recipe, page 193)

Post-Workout

BURN ZONE

Black tea
Coffee
Electrolytes
Small cup of bone broth
Sparkling water
Water
Water with Himalayan pink salt
Zero-calorie electrolyte water

BOOST ZONE

Avocado
Bacon
Broccoli
Celery
Cheese
Cucumber
Eggs
Full-fat yogurt
Grass-fed meat protein bars (see Resources, page 303)
Grilled chicken
Handful of nuts
Jerky
Kale
Olives
Pickles
Protein shake
Spinach
Sprouts
Vegetable smoothie

Week Five and Beyond

This one week of workouts will take you through the initial four weeks of your Cruise Control commitment, but as the weeks continue to roll forward, feel free to shake up your workouts a bit—you can also create your own customized Cruise Control Workout plan by mixing and matching the days in the planner. I suggest taking a few minutes on a Sunday (or any day before kicking off the new week of workouts) to sit down and write out a week's worth of workouts. That way, as the week gets going, you won't have any work to do or any extra "stuff" to think about. Just as I always recommend actually scheduling your eight minutes of workout time into your calendar so you won't have an excuse to miss it, I wholeheartedly believe that having a no-brainer, already developed workout for each day will make it that much easier for you to stick to your workouts.

STEPHANIE **SMITH**

AGE: 30 | WEIGHT LOST: 13 POUNDS

What everyone needs to know: You'll legit choose salads over tacos and enchiladas. I've been a dedicated Cruiser for weeks now, and I love it. I can't believe how much better my stomach looks—even when I'm sitting! My clothes fit amazingly well, my skin is GLOWING, my hair and nails are killing it, and my performance at work is killer. I have so much energy and am sleeping restfully at night. I love Cruise Control!

CHAPTER 9

Healthy Living – Anywhere, Anytime

Take care of your body. It's the
only place you have to live.
— JIM ROHN

S ince each individual is unique, it's impossible to give a
one-size-fits-all prescription for living. I know this from
more than twenty years of working with countless numbers of clients—each and every person has a distinctive
way of moving through the world. We all face different challenges, obstacles, strengths, and places to grow. That's why I've
designed Cruise Control to be a lifestyle you can do anywhere,
anytime, no matter what your circumstances. On the next pages,
you'll find my favorite wellness strategies for Cruising your way
to total health. You'll learn how to do Cruise Control on the go,
what to order when out to eat with friends or family, and which

superfoods and supplements will improve your appearance and quality of life. Cruise Control *is* a one-size-fits-all solution because it is flexible enough to mold to your wants, desires, likes, and dislikes.

Cruise Control is made to shift gears with whatever is going on in your life. Whether you are on the road and forgot to bring food, are staying somewhere with no kitchen, or don't know what to order while dining out—I've got you covered. You'll be on Cruise Control regardless of your circumstances.

NUTRITION

On-the-Go Snacks

When you have time to pack something in your purse, briefcase, bag, or insulated lunch sack, consider these great options.

- Avocado and Himalayan pink salt
- Bacon wrapped in a paper towel
- Celery sticks with almond butter or tahini
- Chomps Meat Sticks (the healthy Slim Jim)
- Dark chocolate bar
- FBOMBs*
- Flax crackers
- Freeze-dried berries
- Fresh berries with whipped coconut milk
- Keto-Snaps and Fat Snax
- Macadamia nuts
- Mixed nuts
- Packets of almond butter or coconut butter
- Parm Crisps or cheese crisps
- Plastic baggies of Benefiber for adding to drinks
- Plastic baggies of collagen peptides for adding to drinks
- Pork rinds
- Pumpkin seeds
- Raw, dry-roasted, smoked almonds

- Seaweed chips
- Tea and/or coffee packets*

*Burn-Zone-Safe

When You Have Time to Pack Snacks

Snacking the Cruise Control way is easy. My favorites have less than a handful of common ingredients that are just thrown together in a bowl and most of them require no cooking.

- Avocado with a squeeze of lemon or lime and salt and pepper
- Bacon-wrapped avocado slices
- Beef jerky
- Celery with nut or seed butter
- Chia Seed Pudding (page 152)
- Cruise Control Coffee (of course, page 143)
- Grass-fed whipped cream with berries
- Hard-boiled eggs
- Jicama with a squeeze of lemon and drizzled with extra-virgin olive oil
- Olives
- Pork rinds
- Pumpkin or sunflower seeds
- Raw almonds, macadamia nuts, or walnuts
- Tea with coconut oil and grass-fed butter

Without a Kitchen

- Avocado
- MCT oil, olive oil, or avocado oil for salads, vegetables, and everything else
- Nut butters
- Nuts
- Single-serve packets of coconut oil
- Snack pack of olives to add to meals or snacks

TRAVEL TIPS

- I never go anywhere without my insulated water bottle. It keeps ice in my water for a full twenty-four hours. I love it.
- If you're stuck with eating out on your trip (because, bummer, you have no kitchen), you can still get plenty of healthy fats by bringing them with you. Online you can find avocado oil, coconut oil, MCT oil, and olive oil in single-serve packets that are easy to carry with you. Plus, they come premeasured. If you don't find them in your grocery store, don't fret—you can order just about any travel-size healthy fat online. See Resources, page 302, for more information.
- Other things I never leave home without are tea bags and coffee packets. It's simple to request hot water whether you are in a hotel lobby or at a restaurant. The packets are also super helpful when you arrive at your destination so that you can make your own Cruise Control Coffee.
- If you're away from home, but you *do* have a kitchen, swing by a local grocery or health food store when you get where you're going to pick up fresh vegetables, meats, and snacks to keep Cruising.

EATING OUT ON CRUISE CONTROL

I travel *a lot* and have frequent business lunches and dinners, which often means I can be eating in restaurants for days at a time. With this in mind, I designed Cruise Control to be friendly to the frequent diner-outer. You won't have any trouble ordering up a Cruise Control–friendly meal no matter where you are eating. Here are some strategies for your next dining-out experience.

DINING TIPS

- You'll find it easier to make substitutions in a fancier restaurant.
- Ask the server to bring your entrées sans potatoes, rice, or other grains.
- Check for gluten-free and grass-fed dairy and meat options.

- Ask for sliced avocados and extra-virgin olive oil in place of other fats.
- Request extra-virgin olive oil and vinegar, lemon, or lime slices for your salad dressing.
- Carry MCT oil, coconut oil, or extra-virgin olive oil packets with you and make your own dressing. Just ask for balsamic vinegar or lemon slices on the side.
- Request beverages such as unsweetened iced teas, hot teas, coffee (hot or iced), and filtered or sparkling water.

MEAL TIPS

- **Greens:** If you have a salad that comes with candied pecans, croutons, or berries or other fruit, request avocado and bacon crumbles as a replacement. Ask for extra-virgin olive oil with vinegar, sliced lemons, or sliced limes. If the oil isn't extra-virgin, skip it.
- **Meats, Poultry, and Fish:** Call around. Many restaurants are now boasting organic, grass-fed, and antibiotic-free beef; choose one of those if possible. Order rich proteins with healthy fats such as salmon, duck, lamb, or pork short ribs. The fattiest steaks are filet mignon, New York strip, T-bone, and rib-eye steaks. However, if the quality of the food is questionable (not antibiotic-free and not organic or free-range), then choose leaner proteins because fat is where toxins are stored.
- **Sushi:** Most sushi places now have a "protein roll" on the menu. If not, just request your sushi without rice, and ask for extra avocado, cucumber, and carrots. While rice alone is super high in carbs, sushi rice is even higher since it's made with sugar and rice vinegar (that's why it tastes so yummy). Finally, skip the rolls with cream cheese, sugary sauces, and tempura-laden sushi concoctions.
- **Diners and Drive-throughs:** In the mood for a burger? Great. Just be sure to go to an establishment that serves real meat. After you've made sure that you're not ordering something full of chemicals and additives, go for a burger wrapped in lettuce as your first choice. If you're splurging on a bun, see if you can

find a place that has a whole-grain or, better yet, gluten-free option. Ask for a side salad instead of fries, please.

- **Poultry:** If you think a chicken or turkey burger is healthier, hold on! Unless it is real chicken or turkey without chemicals or additives, you don't want it. You also don't want batter-dipped or fried "real" chicken. Choose grilled, broiled, or roasted poultry.
- **Italian:** Ask for vegetables (such as arugula, eggplant, spinach, or zucchini) in place of pasta, and make sure that no sugar is added to tomato-based sauces.
- **Latin:** Mexican and Spanish restaurants often serve up chips and salsa, but you can usually request cucumber slices, spicy carrots, or a salad on the side instead. After that, order yourself some carne asada or chicken and ask for a double serving of veggies instead of the rice and beans. You can also ask for guacamole with raw vegetables, and you can order tacos sans tortillas. Just get the insides with extra shredded lettuce.
- **Indian:** Tandoori chicken, meats, and vegetables are your best bet in an Indian restaurant. Tandoori is marinated in yogurt and spices like garlic and ginger and is then baked in a very hot oven. Request fresh sliced veggies or a side salad instead of the naan or samosas. Watch the vegetable-based curries, as they're often packed with high-carb ingredients.
- **Asian:** Be careful because much of Chinese, Thai, and Japanese food serves "candied" meat, and many sauces have sugar in them. Orange chicken one of your favorites? Yep, sorry, that is batter- and sugar-coated. Instead, order steamed veggies, rice, and un-sauced, un-fried meat.
- **Appetizers:** You'll be better off if you can find a place that serves tapas instead of standard appetizer fare, which is usually made up of a batter-dipped, deep-fried onion, potato, or other food. Tapas tend to consist of olives, cheeses, meats, hummus, and vegetables—much more Cruise Control–friendly. And, sorry, but wings are usually coated with either batter or sugar, so unless you can find a healthy version, skip them.

Grocery Shopping on Cruise Control

There are many healthy options available at your grocery stores and at your fingertips. I love Walmart, Target, Costco, Trader Joe's, and, of course, Amazon. Here's the breakdown:

Walmart: I like Walmart because it has a wide variety of Cruise Control–friendly foods. This is always helpful because I don't have the time to make multiple trips to different supermarkets to get groceries. You can also order your groceries from Walmart online, and they'll carry them right to your car. Here's what to look for:

- Great Value Heavy Whipping Cream
- Philadelphia Cream Cheese
- Kerrygold Pure Irish Butter
- Sam's Choice Beef Smoked Sausage
- Hormel Natural Choice Bacon
- Deli Ham & Pepperoni
- Great Value Organic Unsweetened Coconut Flakes
- Fisher Chopped Pecans
- Great Value Pecan Nuts
- Parm Crisps Cheese Crisps
- Nature's Eats Blanched Almond Flour
- Arrowhead Mills Organic Coconut Flour
- Kettle & Fire Bone Broth
- Better Body Organic Coconut Flour
- Swerve Sweetener
- Ghirardelli Unsweetened Chocolate
- Great Value Sugar-Free Syrup
- Primal Kitchen Salad Dressing
- Great Value Organic Coconut Oil
- Heinz No Sugar Ketchup
- G Hughes Sugar-Free BBQ Sauce
- Smucker's Peanut Butter
- Green Giant Riced Cauliflower
- Primal Kitchen Avocado Oil Mayo
- Rao's Marinara Sauce

- Mezzetta Marinara
- Green Giant Zucchini Spirals
- Chosen Foods Avocado Oil
- Stur Water Enhancer
- Carrington Farms Organic Ghee and Organic Coconut Oil & Ghee
- Sam's Choice Organic Vegetable Broth
- Zevia Soda
- Barlean's Flaxseed Oil

Target: Target also has many Cruise Control–friendly foods. Look for these items:

- Cece's Veggie Noodles
- Market Pantry Plain Cream Cheese
- Driscoll's Organic Berries
- Primal Kitchen Collagen Fuel
- Sir Kensington's Organic Mayonnaise
- Zevia Soda
- Archer Farms Asparagus Spears
- Simply Balanced Organic Eggs
- Stur Water Enhancer
- Let's Do Unsweetened Organic Creamed Coconut
- Simply Balanced Organic Coconut Oil
- Simply Balanced Almond Butter
- Simply Balanced Alaskan Sockeye Salmon
- Applegate Organics Roasted Chicken Breast
- Kerrygold Irish Butter
- Hershey's Unsweetened Cocoa
- Simply Balanced Organic Grass-fed Ground Beef
- Market Pantry Pecan Halves
- Califia Farms Pure Black Cold Brew Coffee
- Applegate Naturals No Sugar Added Bacon
- Wholly Guacamole Minis
- Eggland's Best Hard-Cooked Peeled Eggs

Costco: This is another place where you can find lots and lots of Cruise Control–friendly foods. This is a family favorite of ours, especially because they have a fantastic organic selection. Plus, where else can you get all the food you need *and* simultaneously shop for your new smaller-sized clothes to replace your pre-Cruising apparel?

- Universal Bakery Organic Aussie Bites
- Sambazon Organic Acai Superfruit Packs
- Salmon Fillets with Pesto Butter
- A La Carte Organic Spaghetti Squash
- Three Bridges Egg Bites
- Rhythm Superfoods Organic Roasted Kale
- Milton's Craft Bakers Cauliflower Crust Pizza
- ITO EN Unsweetened Matcha Green Tea Powder
- Nature's Touch Fresh Avocado Chunks
- Elan Coconut Noix De Coco Coconut Slices
- Love Beets Organic Cooked Beets
- Grain & Simple Organic Butternut Squash Spirals
- Kirkland Signature Unsalted Mixed Nuts
- Nature's Touch Avocado Chunks
- Don Lee Farms Plant-Based Burgers
- Kirkland Signature Smoked Pulled Pork
- Primal Kitchen Avocado Oil Mayo
- Nature's Intent Organic Chia Seeds
- Premium Selection Organic Riced Cauliflower
- Explore Cuisine Organic Edamame Spaghetti
- Sunrich Organic Chicken Bone Broth
- Kirkland Signature Dry Roasted Macadamia Nuts
- Seeds of Change Organic Quinoa and Brown Rice
- NuttZo Organic Nut and Seed Butter
- The Good Bean Chickpeas
- Good Culture Cottage Cheese
- Kirkland Organic Hard-Boiled Eggs
- Yancey's Fancy Cheese Curds
- Kirkland Signature Organic Quinoa
- Teton Waters Uncured Beef Polish Sausage
- Kirkland Signature Organic Green Tea
- Manitoba Harvest Organic Hemp Hearts

- NuttZo Nut and Seed Butter
- Oberto Trail Mix
- Birch Benders Paleo Pancake and Waffle Mix
- Banza Chickpea Pasta
- Kirkland Signature Organic Hard-Boiled Eggs
- Made Good Granola Minis

Trader Joe's: Trader Joe's has healthier options than many major grocery store chains. Plus, you can actually sample anything in the store! Yep, ANYTHING! I love this amenity. If you see a new food at Trader Joe's that looks like it might make a good Cruise Control addition, just ask one of the crew to let you sample the item. Here are some of my Trader Joe's faves:

- Chile Lime Chicken Burgers
- Crumbled Feta
- Grilled Cauliflower
- Riced Broccoli
- Organic Raw Almonds
- Zucchini Spirals
- Cauliflower Pizza Crust
- Aged Goat Gouda Cheese
- Organic Grass-Fed Ground Beef
- Shaved Brussels Sprouts
- Organic Virgin Coconut Oil
- Whole Cashews
- Carrot Spirals
- Broccoli Florets
- Seasoned Kale Chips
- Turkey Burgers
- Cauliflower & Broccoli Vegetable Patties
- Organic Pitted Kalamon Olives
- Chomps Snack Sticks
- Clarified Butter (Ghee)
- Broccoli & Kale Slaw
- Rockview Heavy Whipping Cream
- Volpi Gourmet Pepperoni

- Kerrygold Butter
- Les Petites Carrots
- Cauliflower Gnocchi

Amazon: Oh man. There's no denying Amazon. Join Amazon Prime, and you'll get most of your foods in one or two days, and many on the same day (no shipping charge)!

- Julian Bakery Organic Paleo Thin Crackers
- Barlean's Flaxseed Oil
- Palmini Pasta
- Cali'flour Foods Pizza Crust
- Swerve Sweetener
- Fat Snax Cookies
- Kettle & Fire Organic Bone Broth
- Parm Crisps Cheese Crisps
- Chomps Grass-Fed Beef Snacks
- LyteLine Electrolyte Water Enhancer
- Crio Bru Coffee
- Primal Kitchen Avocado Oil Mayo
- Primal Kitchen Salad Dressing
- Primal Kitchen Collagen Fuel
- Alkamind Daily Minerals
- Stur Water Enhancer
- One Body One Life Fat Burning Lemonade
- FBOMB Premium Oil and Nut Butter Packets
- Picnik Butter Coffee
- Zevia Soda
- Laird Superfoods
- Pique Tea
- Oberto Lowrey's Bacon Curls
- Quest Nutrition Protein Chips
- EBOOST Spruce Green Juice Powder

SMART FOOD SHOPPING

Here are my favorite tips for saving money while at the grocery store.

- **Don't just stay on the perimeter.** Huh? I know, I'm such a rebel. Here's the thing. The perimeter of the grocery store is still where you'll find the fresh meats, poultry, and fresh veggies and other produce, but it's also often where you'll find the bakery items (let's face it, the food industry knows about the perimeter tip). You'll also miss out on healthy nuts and seeds and frozen veggies and proteins that will help you in a pinch.
- **Grab on-sale meats.** Check your weekly circulars. You can always find lean cuts of meat on sale.
- **Buy coconut oil.** It's cheaper than grass-fed butter, ghee, and cacao butter/oil.
- **Stick to lower-cost nuts and seeds.** Choose pumpkin seeds, flaxseeds, chia seeds, sesame seeds, sunflower seeds, cashews, almonds, and Brazil nuts.
- **Skip prepackaged foods.** Make your own treats instead!
- **Plan on eating similar foods.** Sometimes less choice is better. Stick to your meal plans every week, at least when you're getting started.
- **Be conscious of the food you're buying.** Don't buy things you won't use.
- **Eat seasonally.** Produce that's in season is generally less expensive.
- **Shop at farmers' markets.** Many of them are not certified organic but use organic practices, which means a lower cost to you.
- **Don't get distracted by new food items.** Load up on full-fat proteins, low-carb vegetables, extra-virgin olive oil, and a couple of spices, and you'll be set.

Meal Delivery Services on Cruise Control

Meal delivery has become all the rage as of late, especially if you listen to podcasts. Blue Apron, HelloFresh, Sun Basket, and many more companies are thriving thanks to the fact that most of us have no time to cook from scratch. Just be careful. I think these are great ideas, but do your research to make sure that you can get meals that will follow the Cruise Control credo. Many times you can share your macro preferences (Boost Zone 50 percent fat, 30 percent carbs, 20 percent protein) and have your meals adjusted accordingly. If a bigger company won't do it, you may be able to find a local smaller resource. I use Factor 75 because not only do they use organic and fresh produce, but their meals are so yummy (and healthy thanks to being designed by registered dietitians). Oh, and they've agreed to do Cruise Control Meals. See the Resources section on page 310 to find more information.

Sweeteners on Cruise Control

If you were paying attention throughout this book, you know that you need to try to avoid all sweeteners as much as possible. And that's because your taste buds really do adapt to what you feed them. That means that if you overly sweeten your beverages, or if you eat things with a lot of added sweeteners (protein bars, yogurts, or cereals), your taste buds "forget" what natural sweetness tastes like. But there's good news because your taste buds will also adjust if you cut out the sugar. Over time, you'll love a bowl of unsweetened berries because your taste buds will have adjusted to natural sweetness. Cutting out the sugar also makes other foods taste better, truly. Sugars dampen our whole eating experience. Plus, now that you've been eating the Cruise Control way, you are fat adapted, so you'll notice that you don't crave sugar like you used to— you're welcome. Bottom line is: Try to avoid sugar and other sweeteners as much as possible, and if you do decide to indulge, check that the food is not overly processed, is within your sixteen-hour Boost Zone, and comes from whole food sources (no additives or preservatives).

Okay, I know we're all going to have a treat from time to time, I mean, let's get real. So here's a review of the Cruise Control–friendly sweeteners you can enjoy safely (in moderation). You'll find the brands I use in parentheses below.

ERYTHRITOL

This is a sugar alcohol that's produced by fermenting the sugar from cornstarch, but it isn't the kind of alcohol that causes intoxication! The result is lots of sweetness, but very few calories. Sugar alcohol is broken down in the small intestine. This means that it won't cause the digestive problems that can occur with some other sugar alcohols. However, if you have kidney problems, check with your doctor or dietitian before consuming erythritol.

(Favorite Brand: Swerve)

MONK FRUIT

Monk fruit is a tiny melon that has been cultivated in China for centuries but is just becoming popular here. The sweetener made from this little guy has twenty times the potency of sugar, but it won't spike your insulin, so it's safe for diabetics. You can find it in most health food stores and Asian markets. Look for a pure form or one blended with stevia.

(Favorite Brand: Julian Bakery Pure Monk)

STEVIA

This sweetener is made from leaves of the stevia plant. It comes with no calories and boasts two hundred times the sweetness of sugar. Stevia has been shown to reduce blood pressure and inflammation. I like using alcohol-free liquid stevia.

(Favorite Non-flavored: Stevia in the Raw)
(Favorite Flavored: Stur)

XYLITOL

Another sugar alcohol, xylitol won't raise blood sugar. You can overdo this sweetener, so be cautious. If you experience gut pain after consuming xylitol, you probably ate too much. Your body comes with an enzyme that breaks this sweetener down, but it can take time for your body to adjust. Plus, this sweetener is toxic in dogs, so keep it away from your pets.

(Favorite Brand: Lite & Sweet)

I didn't include sucralose, aspartame, or saccharin and that's no mistake. Synthetic sweeteners like these aren't going to help you with your health. My recommendation? Avoid them completely.

Alcohol on Cruise Control

With alcohol, moderation is key. While there is research that having a drink (*one drink*) occasionally may reduce the risk of coronary heart disease, possibly stroke, and type 2 diabetes, I'm not condoning three glasses of red wine every night in the name of strengthening your heart. It's a luxury. You can reap any benefit that might come from drinking by following Cruise Control. Plus, if you have weight to lose, drinking alcohol may hinder your results. When you drink, your body burns the alcohol even before carbohydrates, protein, or fat. Having a glass of wine a couple of nights a week won't stop fat burning, but it does make your liver work harder, and excessive alcohol will seriously damage your liver and will block fat burning until the alcohol calories are used up. Bottom line: If you don't respond well to alcohol, or you have trouble stopping at one drink, then just don't. Personally, I only have an alcoholic beverage once a week or on special occasions.

Here are the most popular choices:

CHAMPAGNE
Serving Amount: 4 fl. oz. (120 ml)
Calories: 90
Carb Count: 1.6 g
Sugar: Around 1 to 2 g
Best Choices: Look for the words "extra brut," "brut nature," "pas dose," or "dosage zero," for the lowest amounts of sugars.

RED WINE
Serving Amount: 5 fl. oz. (150 ml)
Calories: 125
Sugar: 0.9 g
Best Choices: Dry wines are best. Choose Cabernet Sauvignon, Syrah, Pinot Noir.

WHITE WINE
Serving Amount: 5 fl. oz. (150 ml)
Calories: 65 to 120
Sugar: 1 to 1.4 g
Best Choices: Again, stick with the dry wines. These include Chardonnay, Pinot Blanc, and Sauvignon Blanc.

LIGHT BEER

Serving Amount: 12 fl. oz. (350 ml)
Calories: 104
Sugar: 0.3 to 2 g
Best Choices: Beck's Premier Light, Miller Genuine Draft 64, Bud Select, Coors Light, Michelob Ultra

VODKA, GIN, RUM

Serving Amount: 1 fl. oz. (30 ml)
Calories: 64
Sugar: 0 g
Best Choices: It doesn't matter so much as long as you mix these with zero-calorie mixers such as water, mineral water, lemon or lime juice, or Zevia soda.

Supportive Nutrients

It used to be that I'd tell clients to only rely on nutrition from food as the best way to supplement and nourish the body with the best nutrients. The problem is that we're all getting older. And with age comes some deterioration, and supplements can be a vital addition to help you stay feeling better for much, much longer. Plus, many of our diets have been devoid of nutrients for so long that supplements can help you get back on course with your health a lot faster.

I'm not saying you should shortcut whole foods. Real food that's organic and local whenever possible is always the best first strategy for your best health. That said, here are the supplements I use and those I recommend to my clients, along with the best food sources, and what the supplement contains.

Bone Strength: The best foods for strengthening bones are greens, nuts and seeds, and salmon and sardines. I take Onnit Stron Bone, which contains: strontium, vitamin K2, vitamin E, potassium, copper, manganese, boron, bioperine.

Curcumin: This is a well-known anti-inflammatory that can be added to your diet by using the spice turmeric or taking turmeric as a supplement in capsule form. This can help with body-wide inflammation and pain. I like the brand Organika Curcumin.

Electrolytes: These are important for keeping your body hydrated. You can find them in artichokes, avocados, bone broth, dark leafy greens, gray sea salt, Himalayan pink salt, and salmon. I love the brand Lyte-Line.

Enzymes: These are good for helping prime better digestion. The best food sources are from organic raw apple cider vinegar or lemon juice (before meals). I also like NOW Foods Super Enzymes.

Iodine: This mineral is found in cod, eggs, seaweed, milk, and tuna, and helps your body to produce thyroid hormones, which help to support a healthy metabolism and proper functioning of several organs and tissues, and can also reduce anxiety and depression. I like a brand called Pure Encapsulations Potassium Iodine.

Magnesium: This is a mineral that helps with protein synthesis, muscle and nerve function, blood glucose control, and the regulation of blood pressure. You can find magnesium in avocados, dark chocolate, dark leafy greens, fish, nuts, and seeds. I like the brand Natural Vitality. Magnesium can also help with sleep, and it is best taken before bed.

Multivitamin: Multivitamins have gotten a bad rap in the news lately, but I still believe that there are good brands, such as Rainbow Light Women's Multi and Men's Multi. Even the most health-motivated client I meet doesn't eat a perfect diet, so a multivitamin is just good health insurance.

Niacin (Vitamin B$_3$): Niacin is one of many B vitamins that helps your body to convert foods you eat into energy you can use. You can find niacin in avocado, beef, chicken, liver, mushrooms, pork, salmon, and turkey. I recommend NOW Foods Flush-Free Niacin.

Omega-3: This type of fatty acid has been shown to improve memory, arthritis pain, heart health, cholesterol numbers, to reduce some cancers, and to lower high blood pressure. You can find these fatty acids in grass-fed beef, Brussels sprouts, cauliflower, flaxseeds, salmon, sardines, shrimp, and walnuts. I like the brand Alkamind Daily Omega-3.

Probiotics: These help to promote the good bacteria in your gut. You can find them in kefir, kimchi, sauerkraut, and sour pickles. I recommend Organifi Biotic Balance Probiotic 50 billion CFU's.

Selenium: This essential mineral helps to fight oxidative stress and to boost antioxidants in the body. You can find it in grass-fed beef, Brazil nuts, cod, chicken, lamb, oysters, salmon, sardines, scallops, sunflower seeds, and turkey. I like the brand Onnit ViruTech.

Vitamin A: This fat-soluble vitamin helps to preserve your vision, body growth, immune function, and fertility. You can find it in cod liver oil, egg yolks, grass-fed butter, and liver. I recommend Barlean's Cod Liver Oil.

Vitamin B Complex: B-vitamins help turn your food into nutrients your body can use to produce energy. Many B-vitamins can be found in dark leafy greens, chicken, and some seafood. I recommend Onnit Active B Complete.

Vitamin B$_{12}$: This vitamin helps to keep your nervous system and blood cells balanced and healthy. It also improves energy and stamina. You can find it in grass-fed beef, eggs, and some brands of milk. I like the brand Life Extension Vitamin B12. If you are interested in B_{12} injections, request methylcobalamin because it is the best absorbed and retained.

Vitamin C: We are lucky because vitamin C is abundant in many foods, such as bell peppers, broccoli, chilies, kale, strawberries, and tomatoes. This vitamin helps to form collagen, improves iron absorption, improves immunity, helps your body heal wounds, and helps maintain your bones. I like the brand LivOn Labs Lypo-Spheric Vitamin C.

Vitamin D: Nicknamed the sunshine vitamin because your body produces vitamin D when exposed to the sun, this vitamin builds strong bones by helping your body to absorb calcium and phosphorus. There is also some evidence that vitamin D can help with reducing some forms of cancer and also depression. You can find vitamin D in cod liver oil, egg yolks, liver, mushrooms, salmon, and sardines, but the best source of vitamin D is what you'll get after 10 to 15 minutes in natural sunlight. I like the brand Onnit Vitamin D3 Spray with Vitamin K2 in MCT Oil.

Vitamin K2: This vitamin is found in broccoli, Brussels sprouts, cauliflower, greens, and grass-fed butter, grass-fed meats, and cheese and eggs from grass-fed animals as well. I like the brand Life Extension Super K with Advanced K2 Complex.

Vitex: The fruit and seed of this plant are commonly taken as a supplement for PMS (premenstrual syndrome) symptoms and to improve fertility and breast health. I like the brand Nature's Way Vitex Fruit.

Zinc: This mineral helps to shorten the duration of colds and improves the function of your immune system. You can find it in eggs, cashews, grass-fed beef, and pumpkin seeds. I recommend NOW Foods Zinc.

NAVIGATING ROADBLOCKS

Finally, let's take a look at life's roadblocks. Even the most perfectly structured and uncomplicated life is still, well, life. And as we all know, life comes with opportunities to grow, and let's face it, challenges, issues, and obstacles that can trip you up. Here are the most common and the Cruise Control solutions to each.

Sleep

We used to think that sleep was simply a time when we rested, but there's so much more going on. Today we know that sleep is when your body is focusing on repair and rejuvenation of all the cells in your brain and body. A lack of sleep throws off your body's balance in myriad ways while getting your quota of sleep helps you to lose weight, stay at a healthy weight, lower stress, improve memory, reduce heart disease, reduce high blood pressure, and reduce the risk of diabetes and stroke. While you consciously do your work during the day to keep your body and brain healthy, when you sleep your body and brain take over and process all that you've done during the day to get you ready to thrive tomorrow. It's pretty amazing, and you don't want to mess around with your snooze time. Aim to get eight hours every night. Here's how to build up your sleep habit:

Close the Kitchen

After your last Boost meal or snack, shut your kitchen for the night. You can have one counter where you set out your Burn Zone supplies to make decaf tea or coffee, but close all the rest for the night. Sticking to a strict Burn Zone will help you to lose more weight, even if you eat more during the day. According to researchers at the Salk Institute, when they had mice either follow a sixteen-hour fasting schedule (which is what you'll be doing in the Burn Zone) or eat whenever they wanted, the mice who didn't eat at night stayed lean, while the twenty-four-hour nibblers got fat.

Create a Sanctuary

The best sleep environment is tranquil, quiet, and dark—extremely dark. This means you need to shut off all screens and devices. When Oxford University investigators followed subjects' sleep patterns, they found that those who had the darkest rooms to sleep in were more than 20 percent less likely to be overweight or obese when compared to those who slept in the lightest bedrooms. The dark at night helps your brain to produce your sleep hormone melatonin and reduces hormones that keep you awake, such as cortisol and adrenaline.

This affects our kids, too. There are numerous studies that show that the kids who are vegging out on TVs, video games, tablets, smartphones, or laptops are more likely to be overweight or obese. In another study, parents of 234 children ages eight to seventeen were surveyed about the hours their kids spent on screens of one type or another. The findings, not surprisingly, were that those kids who had the most exposure to screens slept less and were more likely to be overweight or obese.

If you read on an iPad or Kindle, turn the light down low. If you are going to use your phone or laptop, look for a night feature in Settings. Get cozy, and use your room only to sleep at bedtime and for intimate time with your spouse. All other activities are best done in other rooms.

Give Your Bed a Makeover

If you have tried all the other methods of creating a sleep haven, but you still have trouble sleeping, analyze your bed. I recommend using 100 percent natural cotton sheets, replacing your pillows about once every year and a half, and making sure that your blankets are made from allergy-free materials. Many of the newer über-soft blankets that are now available are made of 100 percent polyester. These can exacerbate premenopausal symptoms such as hot flashes and night sweats. Finally, check your mattress. I know. Mattresses are expensive. It's true, but this is one place where I truly believe you can't skimp. Cheaper mattresses can be filled with all sorts of chemicals and materials that can disrupt your sleep. Do your research. I've been really happy with my Samina mattress (see Resources, page 316, for more information). Some even have petrochemical foams that give off completely odor-free but toxic fumes.

Add a Chill

You'll sleep better if your room is a little on the chilly side. It seems that we like to hibernate just like bears when it gets cold, according to research presented at a joint meeting of endocrine experts. Not only that, but the researchers found that sleeping in colder rooms also helps you to burn belly fat while you sleep. Published in the journal *Diabetes*, this study found that colder sleeping environments help enhance the effectiveness of our stores of brown fat—brown fat is easier for your body to burn than white fat—and it's especially helpful in the burning of belly fat. The best temperature? Around 66 degrees. Sleeping in rooms that were 75 to 81 degrees didn't work as well. After four weeks of sleeping in the coldest rooms, the subjects in the study almost doubled their volumes of fat-burning brown fat, and these subjects lost belly fat as well.

Soak Your Way to Sleep

Another way to make your room feel colder is to take a warm bath or shower about an hour and a half before you want to go to sleep. Soaking in or under the warmth of water causes your body temperature to rise, and then giving yourself time before bed will allow your temperature to naturally drop. This is a modern way of encouraging your body to first heat up and then cool down. This little trick can "help" your body to release sleep hormones and decrease stress hormones. When humans lived mostly outdoors, this natural heating and cooling of the body would happen in accordance with the day, but in our hyper climate-controlled indoor habitats, that doesn't often occur.

Loosen Up

You'd fall asleep faster if you had a nightly massage. Studies show that massage helps trigger the release of serotonin, a neurotransmitter that can enhance the feeling of tranquillity. Duh. But who has the time and money for that? Even if you can't ask or cajole your partner into giving your shoulders or legs a little massage, you can still decrease anxiety and improve sleep quality with self-massage. You can use a simple tennis ball to roll on sore muscles, or there are several gadgets you can find online. I like to use one called the MyoBuddy Massager Pro because it gives what feels like a deep-tissue massage, and it's heated. See Resources, page 314, for more information and options.

Have a Set Bedtime

Another thing that helps melatonin (the sleep hormone) come out at night is to have a set bedtime. It's best to schedule bedtime to occur around three hours after your last Boost Zone meal or snack. According to Dr. Panda from the Salk Institute, this helps your digestive system and other systems in your body to get the message that it's bedtime, and helps it switch to repair and replenish mode. Just as your body will come to "expect" certain foods at certain times, it will come to expect your bedtime and wake time to occur on a schedule.

Keep a Notepad Handy

Having paper and pen within arm's reach of your bed will give you a handy place to put down any leftover worries, obligations, errands, and other thoughts that can keep you up at night. You'll be able to rest and relax better after putting thoughts on paper (and getting them out of your head), so you can let go of the day's stress and not worry about what's on tomorrow's schedule.

Have a Nighttime Tea

Have a Cruise Control Tea made with decaf chai or rooibos tea. Chai is made with Ayurvedic herbs that settle and clean your digestive system, and rooibos has a powerful flavonoid called aspalathin, which has been shown to reduce stress hormones that trigger hunger and fat storage.

Track Your Snooze Time

There are plenty of apps available on smartphones that track sleep and wake times. If you already believe you are getting enough sleep, but you are struggling with excess weight, start to track your sleep closely. You can also do this on your handy notepad. Jot down when you go to sleep, any nighttime awakenings, and your morning wake-up time. If you have a restless night, note what happened during the previous day. Did you exercise? Drink too much coffee or caffeine? Have a stressful time at work? Ate too much food too late into the evening? Look for patterns. Use what you discover so you can tweak and alter your daytime activities to better support your sleep.

TIPS FOR DAYTIME ALERTNESS

The Cruise Control Diet is designed to convert your body from being a sugar burner to a fat burner. During this process, you may experience some initial tiredness or fatigue. But the good news is that this is only temporary. As your body relies less on sugar and more on fat for energy, these symptoms will go away. Here are my top tips for overcoming fatigue:

- Drink a cup of Cruise Control Coffee.
- Have a cup of green tea (it has powerful antioxidants that boost your energy levels).
- Do some simple stretches to activate your body and mind.
- Go outside and get some vitamin D.
- Stay hydrated and make sure you are getting enough water.

WEIGHT PLATEAUS

One of the best parts of Cruise Control is that plateaus are much less likely than on other diets. Still, if you find that you go through a few days or a week where you do not see any changes on the measuring tape or scale, don't give up. A plateau is perfectly normal and very often will resolve itself on its own. Rest assured that you are still in the fat-burning zone and the scale will start moving soon. A plateau is considered three consecutive days without weight loss. Possible reasons include:

- Stress
- Menstrual cycle

- Eating too few or too many calories
- Exposure to pesticides, chemicals, and toxins from nonorganic foods
- Lack of sleep
- Consuming foods not included on the Cruise Control Shopping List

If you hit a plateau and do not experience any weight loss by the fourth day, it's time to reroute and reinvigorate your weight loss. Obviously, if you have been indulging in some non–Cruise Control foods, recommit and start again. In addition, you can try one of the following rerouting measures:

- **Skip the fruit:** Take a day off having one or both servings of fruit, and you can replace this with one tablespoon of coconut oil, macadamia nut oil, avocado oil, or extra-virgin olive oil.
- **Eliminate snacks:** Only consume two Boost Zone Meals and your Burn Zone treats each day.
- **Extend your burn:** Cut your Boost Zone to six hours for a few days, and do an eighteen-hour Burn Zone.
- **Try a probiotic:** These supplements can rebalance your gut and help your intestines to be better at eliminating wastes and toxins.

STRESS

We live in an overly stressed society of people who live with a 24/7 plugged-in mentality. To de-stress means that you need to *unplug*, to disengage from life's to-do list. Here are my favorite strategies for when I'm feeling overly wound up or just overwhelmed.

Move

Doctors tend to agree that exercise is one of the best forms of medicine out there: a boost of endorphins leaves you feeling calm and energized and will boost your mood while lowering your stress. Research has shown that regular exercise can reduce depression and stress as well as prescription meds. Try to get some movement in your life every day. See chapter 8 for more tips on staying active.

Meditate

It works. Researchers from Harvard and McGill conducted a review of twenty-nine stress-reducing meditation studies (including more than twenty-five hundred subjects) and found that meditation had the greatest effect on reducing stress, and also reduced depression, distress, anxiety, and burnout.

Anyone can and should meditate. Here's how: There's no need to go to a Buddhist monastery or on a silent retreat, although both might be cool to experience. You can meditate anywhere and anytime, even for just a few minutes. Meditating just means bringing your mind's awareness into the present. The most common way to do this is to focus on your breathing, but you can also focus on sounds, sights, and feelings. Example: Instead of going into autopilot while washing the dishes, bring your mind's attention to exactly what you are doing. Slow down. Feel the warm soapy water, look at each dish or cup you wash, and wash slowly and methodically. Mindfully focusing on the dishes *is* meditating. Alternatively, have a seat. Anywhere that's quiet. Set your timer to five minutes. Get comfy. Bring your attention to your breathing. Focus on each inhale and exhale. When your mind wanders (and it will because that's what minds are made to do), notice it and bring your attention back to your breath. Get it?

Even if you feel like you are horrible at meditating, that your mind is always wandering, it doesn't matter. Each time you notice a wandering mind and bring it back to the present, you've succeeded. And, whether you feel it or not, you've lowered any overly aggravated stress hormones and increased your feel-good neurotransmitter, serotonin. You can do the same thing by sitting and listening to whatever sounds are going on—everything can be part of awareness, and awareness lowers stress. Still need help? My all-time favorite app is the Insight Timer. You'll find bazillions of choices for free on this app. There are also Calm, Headspace, and many other meditation apps. Do a search and see what you like. Try to meditate once a day for at least five minutes.

Balance Your Breathing

Deep and slow breathing activates your body's calming response, lowers levels of inflammation, and releases tension and stress.

I love Dr. Andrew Weil's recommendation for breathing—the famous, relaxing 4-7-8 method. It's simple: You inhale slowly to the count of four, pause and hold your breath at the top for seven seconds, and then exhale slowly to the count of eight. Most people forget the "slow" part, which can lead to trouble. If you breathe deeply but quickly, you can set off anxiety signals in your brain and cause hyperventilation. Also, be sure to exhale fully. That's why it gets the most seconds from Dr. Weil. This is an important method to remove toxins from your body, and most of us don't exhale fully enough. Try the 4-7-8 now. As you inhale, push your belly out to a slow count of four, hold at the top for seven seconds, and as you exhale, your belly should come in toward your spine.

If you're ever stuffed up with allergies or a cold and you are having trouble breathing, be cautious of using nasal sprays. Many can cause rebound reactions that get you stuck in a cycle of constantly clogged nasal passages. I try to stay natural by just using a saline rinse or spray. The one I like to use is called Xlear because it is entirely free of addictive or rebound reactions. Xlear is made with saline and xylitol and is great at clearing and moisturizing sinuses. I use this to help me sleep at night and before a workout to breathe better. You can find more information about where to buy it in the Resources section, page 312.

Perfect Your Posture

The way you sit and stand affects how you feel. Don't believe it? Try this: The next time you are in a group setting, notice how you are feeling. Are you sitting hunched over? Arms and legs crossed? Is your body curled up? Alternatively, are you sitting up? Is your body open? Notice how you feel. Research shows that sitting upright helps you reduce stress and improves confidence, creates a better mood, and lowers fear to boot. Try it out. If you notice you are "sitting small," open up your arms, roll your shoulders down and back, sit up, lift your head so you are looking straight forward, and uncross your legs. You'll notice your stress melting away, and you'll feel empowered, self-confident, and positive.

Get Outside

We spend 87 percent of our lives indoors. If you add in the time we are in our autos, it jumps to more than 95 percent! Walking outside for any amount of time gives your body exposure to nature and sunlight. Even a few trees will do. Studies show that exposure to nature relieves stress and depression, and so does sunlight (even on a rainy day). Focusing on nature (plants, trees, flowers, birds, squirrels) relaxes your mind because your brain associates these things with tranquillity. The response is a nice balancing of your stress and happy hormones. There's something magical about exercising outside, or even just strolling, that you can't get in a gym. Research shows that a ninety-minute stroll in nature will lower the pessimistic part of your brain—it will make you feel happier and more relaxed.

You don't have to do it all in one chunk of time. Try this: On your lunch break, walk to the park. Don't forget to carry your Cruise Control lunch with you. Sit on a park bench and eat your Boost Zone meal and walk back. That's going to cover around an hour outside. Then in the evening or morning, get outside to walk your dog, water some plants, play with your kids, wash your windows, or even clean your car. You'll feel better. I promise. If you are stuck inside, at least look at some pictures of a trip you took when you *were* in a beautiful place in nature. Research shows that this can also help lower stress.

Practice Self-Care

Taking time out for yourself is important. Self-care also includes setting aside time to practice basic daily but nurturing life activities such as washing and moisturizing your face to cleanse away all the toxins of the day, brushing and flossing your teeth, and a weekly deep moisturizer for your hair and skin-rejuvenating mask for your face. Don't forget to get a mani-pedi, either! For even deeper rejuvenation, there's a new self-care product that I love called NanoVi (see Resources on page 316 for more information). This futuristic little machine delivers a fine mist that has been powered up in a way that helps your cells repair and rejuvenate to improve mental and physical performance, speed recovery from workouts, and increase energy (see "My Fifteen-Minute Secret," page 265). Plus, it's easy to use.

Be Grateful

One of my favorite quotes is: "Need a reason to be grateful? Check your pulse." I don't know who said it, but it reminds me that there's always something to be grateful for in my life. Clean sheets, stocked fridge, beautiful kids, loving husband. Taking notice (on paper is best) of at least five things a day that you are grateful for will help recalibrate your mind for less negativity and greater happiness. Gratitude tricks you into feeling more positive because you are taking notice of good experiences, cherished people, and positive circumstances. This helps you to deal with adversity, lowers stress, and improves self-confidence. Gratitude has been shown to lower the stress hormone cortisol around 23 percent. Plus, you'll sleep better, be more energized, and lower your inflammation, according to a study by researchers at the University of California, San Diego's School of Medicine.

Get Lit

No, not with booze. Alcohol actually exacerbates stress. I'm talking about light. I know I already plugged going outside as a tip, but while natural light is great, not all of us are lucky enough to live in a climate where it's always sunny. Natural sunlight is a great way to boost your mood and lower stress, but so are lights that use bulbs that mimic natural light. Plus, these lights can be combined with many of the strategies above for lowering stress, such as mindful thinking, meditating, and writing a gratitude list. For a triple threat strike at unhealthy, toxic stress, you can do all three. There's also a certain type of light you can use when you are getting ready to go to sleep, which sounds weird but is true. Dr. Satchin Panda, circadian rhythm researcher at the Salk Institute in San Diego, says it's best to sleep in a completely dark room, but he also doesn't expect everyone to go sit in a dark room in the evenings before bed. Instead, Panda suggests using table lamps that reduce the amount of blue light by using dim table lamps instead of bright overhead lights.

STEP INTO THE LIGHT FOR LESS STRESS AND BETTER HEALTH

I'm always searching for new ways to upgrade my health, and I love finding technology hacks that help to improve it. For the last few years, I've been using a light therapy device called Joovv (see Resources, page 315, for more information) to resync my body's clock to help me reduce stress, sleep better, and feel more energized during the day. I sleep better, have less stress, and recover from workouts faster. Your body is designed to be in sync with the sun. But today, the average American spends 93 percent of the time indoors, and most of that time is spent surrounded by artificial light. Modern living means spending far too many hours under the glow of computers, phone, tablets, bright overhead lights, and TV screens. These lights and screens hit us with blue light, which has been shown to disrupt sleep, increase stress, and deplete energy and can cause headaches, eye strain, and sleepless nights.

The red light therapy boxes I found are space friendly and come in different sizes. After about ten minutes under red light, I feel my tension melt away. I also can feel relief in achy joints and muscles. According to research, these red light boxes have been shown to stimulate the mitochondria (your energy chargers) in your cells and fight against the bad guys (nitric oxide and oxidative stress) that clog up your body's ability to make energy from food and nutrients. Light therapy has also been shown to boost mood, improve thyroid health, aid weight loss, and boost testosterone in men.

MY FIFTEEN-MINUTE SECRET

What if there were a machine you could use to help you mentally and physically recover and regenerate faster and better? I know. I'd want one, too. Here's the good news. It exists! There's a machine that you can have in your home to repair and regenerate your body at a cellular level. The NanoVi is used to improve mental and physical performance, accelerate repair and recovery, and increase energy. Find out more in the Resources section, page 316. The company has made its technology available to human studies, and, in the process, findings have shown positive improvement in cellular DNA repair, improved immune response, and increased balance in the nervous system. This not only helps you to recover from workouts with less soreness, but NanoVi reduces stress and increases vitality. A side benefit to the NanoVi is that it is enjoyable to use. It feels like breathing in a cool mist. I can do it while I'm answering emails, watching a movie, reading a book, or even taking a business call. My clients love the NanoVi.

DEALING WITH DETOX SYMPTOMS

Detox reactions can occur during the Cruise Control program. In most cases, they appear as minor headaches, fatigue, or occasional loose bowels or slowed elimination. This will typically occur during the first five to seven days of the program. Detox reactions, while no fun, are often an indicator that your system is shifting to the positive. For example, if you have been drinking diet or regular sodas, smoking cigarettes, and consuming processed foods, your body will need a little time to adjust to your new, healthy lifestyle. Be gentle with yourself and just take it one day at a time. Soon you'll be feeling fantastic.

Hunger: This is probably the most commonly voiced concern Cruisers mention when they start out on the eight-to-sixteen-hour Boost to Burn

Zone. You might assume that you will be overwhelmed with hunger, especially in the Burn. That's not how it works. We've been taught to fear hunger, but it really isn't something that persists endlessly. Hunger occurs in waves. If you do experience hunger, know that it will pass. Staying busy is often helpful at first. When your body becomes accustomed to Cruise Control, it will switch from burning sugar (glucose) to burning fat. When this happens, the feelings of hunger are suppressed. Fat is a long and slow-burning fuel, while sugars burn like lighter fluid. In fact, most of my clients say that their appetites don't increase on Cruise Control—they decrease!

Dizziness: If you experience dizziness you are probably dehydrated, and you may also be low on electrolytes. You can easily remedy this by adding a pinch of Himalayan pink salt to a glass of water, a cup of bone broth, or a cup of tea. Another possibility is that you have low blood pressure, especially if you're on hypertension medication. If you have concerns, talk to your doctor.

Headaches: During your first few days of adjusting to Cruise Control, you may have a headache. It might be that you just need that pinch of salt in water, broth, or tea that I mentioned above. Even though highly processed and sugary items are bad for your health, cutting them out can cause headaches (it's just your body detoxifying itself).

Bowel Movements: Ideally, you want to have one to two regular and easy bowel movements each day (usually at around the same time each day). Cruisers don't typically have any trouble with pooping. If your gut flora is at a proper level, you shouldn't have a problem with your body cleansing itself naturally. Reduction in normal bowel movements can be, but is not always, the same as constipation. Constipation is characterized by stool that has a hard consistency and often requires straining and is difficult to pass, but it's unlikely on Cruise Control. Why? The Burn Zone foods and treats keep your system flowing, *and* the Boost Zone meals are full of fiber to keep your gut scrubbed clean. When you lose weight, regardless of the diet you follow, a lot of that will be waste that has built up inside your body. It may be that you have some built-up waste in your intestines. Check your tummy. Is the padding on your belly flabby or firm? I call the firm stuff "false belly fat." This is most likely a buildup of fecal matter (poop) that is stuck to the walls of your intestines. This is especially common among people who eat lots of overly processed products—junk food gums up your pipes! (Gross, right?)

Don't panic. You'll soon be flushing waste like a champ thanks to the abundance of plant-based, fiber-rich, and healthy-fat-filled meals, snacks, and beverages you're going to Burn and Boost on Cruise Control. If you still have issues, you can add a fiber supplement, or you can take a daily probiotic for extra gut support. Look for a probiotic with at least 10 billion active cultures.

Heartburn: If you suffer from indigestion, sour stomach, or heartburn after the Burn Zone, eat a smaller meal when you break your Burn. During the Boost Zone, avoid lying down immediately after a meal. Staying in an upright position for at least a half hour after a meal can help improve your digestive cycle. If you find yourself with a bad case of heartburn, drink a cup of water with a teaspoon of baking soda mixed in.

Muscle Cramps: Diabetics are often low in magnesium, and this can cause muscle cramps. You may take an over-the-counter magnesium supplement, but first, try to bulk up on magnesium-rich foods. These include leafy green vegetables, pumpkin seeds, and Brazil nuts. Another great, enjoyable way to boost magnesium is to take a bath with an added cup of Epsom salts—the magnesium will be absorbed through your skin.

Stiff Muscles: Stretching loosens muscles and encourages deep breathing. Aim to stretch for at least five to ten minutes if you have stiff muscles. Using a foam roller is one of the most effective ways to loosen stiff muscles. Stretching after waking, before bedtime, or both will also help alleviate tight muscle groups and improve flexibility!

IMPROVING INTIMACY ON CRUISE CONTROL

I know. You're overwhelmed, stressed, trying to lose weight, and fit in work and exercise, so maybe sex is the last thing on your mind. You are not alone. Depression, anxiety, medications, health issues, and depleted sex hormones reduce desire in the bedroom for most people. Long before menopause, around 40 percent of women experience a reduced libido. Usually, we only think of testosterone as the sex hormone in men, but women have testosterone, too. The good news is that certain foods will ramp up your libido by increasing your blood flow, balancing and increasing sex hormones, and improving desire-building endorphin highs in your brain and body. Below are your best bets.

- **Pumpkin Seeds:** According to Dr. Mehmet Oz, zinc is the ultimate sex mineral because it helps to boost levels of testosterone (it's not just for us guys, ladies). Your body produces testosterone as well as estrogen and progesterone, and all three decrease and fluctuate as you age. These little green seeds are rich in zinc. A quarter cup for a snack any time of the day—Boost or Burn—can help your hormones get back into balance.
- **Greens:** Magnesium, a mineral, increases blood flow by reducing inflammation in blood vessels (giving them more room to better circulate blood). Better circulation helps your extremities get better blood flow, which can increase arousal in men and women and make sex more pleasurable.
- **Green Tea:** I've talked a lot about tea, but there's something special about the green stuff. Green tea is especially rich in compounds called catechins, which have other belly- and body-fat-burning abilities, but they also boost desire by promoting blood flow *down there*. Blood flow to your genitals helps you feel sexual arousal, so sipping the stuff is actually sexier than red wine.
- **Seafood:** Doesn't sound very sexy, does it? But omega-3 fatty acids increase your heart health and raise dopamine levels in your brain. The result is better circulation and blood flow, which can trigger arousal. You'll feel more connected and relaxed. Your best bets are salmon and tuna.

- **Dark Chocolate:** There's a reason chocolate became a gift given before amorous activity. Dark chocolate (70 percent or more cocoa) increases dopamine levels (your pleasure chemical), and this yummy stuff also opens up blood vessels and improves blood flow. Plus, dark chocolate increases levels of the mood-boosting neurotransmitter serotonin, which can lower stress levels, boosting desire and making it easier to reach orgasm.
- **Garlic:** This pungent little bulb has mighty sex powers. Garlic contains a compound that thins your blood, which improves circulation. Garlic helps stop the formation of new fatty deposits that can clog up your arterial walls and decrease circulation.

MAURA COYLE

AGE: 46 | WEIGHT LOST: 13 POUNDS

What everyone needs to know: Cruise Control will change your mind. Here are just some of the things my mind was telling me before I started Cruising:

"I don't have willpower, and I'll never lose weight. I can't make this life change. I don't have time to plan healthy meals or buy healthy stuff. I can't find time to work out. I can't put butter in my coffee and like it. I can't go sixteen hours without eating. I can't stand up to people who don't support me. I can't drink THAT MUCH water. I can't socialize without drinking and eating. I won't lose weight eating that much fat or be able to exercise without more carbs. I won't ever like what I see in the mirror."

Guess what?

My mind lied. I'm as surprised as you are, but Cruise Control has taught me to shut down the negative and to trust in the positive. Today I got dressed for work, and my skin felt nice and tight, I turned to look at my reflection, and I felt truly happy.

CHAPTER 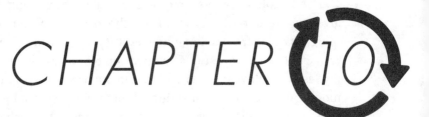10

You've Got Questions, I've Got Answers

'I've taught my Cruise Control Diet to countless clients and online Cruisers and so I've fielded my fair share of questions about it. This chapter answers the most common questions I get.

FASTING WORRIES

Won't my body go into starvation mode when I fast?

Starvation mode—the scary kind where your belly gets bloated, and you die—is not something that happens in sixteen hours. It doesn't even happen in several days. To truly go into starvation mode, you would need to have severely reduced access to food for months. That said, factually speaking, any time you restrict calories you put your body in a sort of "starvation mode," but this isn't the sort of calorie debt that is dangerous to your body. Remember that back in the Paleolithic era it was common for people to go several days without food. You are biologically set up to deal with this lack of energy by burning the fat you have in your stores.

When it comes to modern-day dieting, you've probably heard the warnings that if you cut your food intake too low, your body will panic and cause you to be overly hungry and to have intense cravings, which will eventually lead you to overeat. Or maybe you've heard that if you cut calories too dramatically and lose weight too fast, your body will greedily hang on to any calories that you do get from food; that any weight you lose will quickly pile back on your body when you finally give in and eat. Or maybe you've heard that starvation mode is when your body slows down your metabolism in response to lack of food. That doesn't happen, either. In fact, your metabolism actually speeds up during fasting because more complicated biological processes have to take place for your body to burn fat. The problem today, for the vast majority of us, isn't starving—it's being chronically *over*fed.

Will fasting burn up my muscle tissue?

If you fast, you'll burn fat, not muscle. Your body is a magnificent and intelligent machine that is biologically engineered to survive periods of time when food is scarce. One of the main reasons we store our food as body fat is so it is available when food is not. Muscle is made of much more complex and tightly wound proteins that are not easily accessible to your body. Only in the most dire circumstances, when your overall body fat drops below 4 percent, will your body begin to use muscle for fuel. One study that tracked weight loss in obese adults found that alternate-day fasting for more than two months resulted in weight loss of up to 8 percent and fat loss of more than 10 percent, but muscle and bone density remained unchanged.

As you begin to incorporate the Cruise Control Burn and Boost Zones, your body will increase its ability to burn fat automatically. At the same time, burning protein for fuel will actually decrease. When you don't eat for a period of time, your body is actually triggered to conserve muscle.

Here's another thing that happens—you lose extra flabby skin! It's truly amazing. I learned this when I was talking to Dr. Jason Fung, author of *The Complete Guide to Fasting*. "People think that when you fast [or Burn] that you'll lose muscle, but you actually lose some unnecessary protein and fat," says Fung. Why would you want to lose protein? Because that's what all that extra skin is made from, and sticking with a committed Burn/Boost Zone results in that excess protein going away. Your body can actually use it as fuel. Cruisers who have lost a substantial amount of weight tell me that they notice loose skin tightening up and wrinkles becoming less noticeable. Fung says that obese people carry anywhere from 20 to 50 percent more protein on their bodies than a healthy-weight person. Remember that the Burn and Boost Zones are designed to signal your body to burn fat preferentially instead of muscle.

Will I get low blood sugar when I fast?

One of the first things people do if they feel shaky or dizzy is to assume that they need to have a spoonful of honey or a glass of orange juice because their blood sugar must be too low. This isn't how your blood sugar works. Remember, your master hormone, insulin, keeps a tight watch on your blood sugar and many other biological mechanisms that work to keep your blood sugar within a healthy range. During the time of day that you don't eat, your body breaks down glycogen (remember that's the glucose that is in your liver for short-term energy), which happens every night when you sleep.

Won't I end up overeating during the Boost Zone?

Studies that look at fasting *do* indicate that your calorie intake does increase the day after you haven't had any food. But if you look at simple math, it's easy to see that it doesn't begin to cover the calories you didn't have the day before. On the day after a one-day fast, according to one study, your average caloric intake increases about 400 calories. Do the math. Let's say that on a normal day you'd eat 2,000 calories, so the day after a fast you eat 2,400 calories. If you add up the average number of calories for two days without fasting you'd have 4,000 calories or 2,000 average per day. With a day of fasting, you have 2,400 for those same forty-eight hours or an average of 1,200 a day. The increased calories don't come close to making up for the lack of calories on the fasting day. On Cruise Control I see the opposite effect. My experience with hundreds of clients shows that, over time, appetite naturally decreases after the sixteen-hour Burn Zone.

Doesn't fasting cause my metabolism to slow down?

First of all, this isn't fasting, but even if it were, you wouldn't shut down your metabolism. You'd actually accelerate it. The same thing happens in the Burn Zone. Think about it. Our human ancestors would never have survived into the modern era. Those hunter/gatherers were out seeking animals for dinner and foraging the forest for vegetables and herbs. They didn't wake up to a tray of doughnuts and a steaming vanilla latte. These nomads needed to have a revved metabolism, especially on the days that food was scarce, so they could chase the prey when they found it. You are biologically designed to rev up your metabolic functions, especially when your insulin is low—and it will be super low in the Burn Zone because you'll be burning powerful fat from your stores. Our ancestors' pattern of feasting and fasting, similar to the Burn and Boost Zones, also preserves muscle mass. Of course, if you try to live on blueberry muffins, energy bars, shakes, and skinny vanilla lattes, your metabolism will slow down. Why? Your insulin will be constantly spiked, and so you'll constantly crave more, while your body will be told to take the calories you eat and turn them into fat. That won't be the reality on Cruise Control—you'll eat delicious food, and plenty, within the Boost *and* Burn Zones.

Will I become nutrient-deficient?

During the Cruise Control Boost and Burn Zones, you'll provide your body with superior nutrient-packed meals that will contain all the vitamins, minerals, proteins, fats, and carbohydrates your body could want. There will be no time for nutrient deficiency on Cruise Control because my menu planners are set up to put you on autopilot to nutrition.

Besides, it is impossible to become carbohydrate deficient, because there is no minimum set amount of carbs you need in your diet. This is not the case with proteins and fats, but I've got you covered. You'll get all the essential amino acids (the building blocks of proteins) and fatty acids to keep you in peak performance on Cruise Control. In fact, by having a daily sixteen-hour Burn Zone, you'll signal your body to keep nutrients instead of excreting them.

CRUISING FAQS

Can I eat as often as I want during the Boost Zone?

Yep! You can eat what you like, whenever you feel like it in your eight-hour Boost Zone. Are you craving a big lunch *and* a big dinner—go for it. Or if you want to graze through your Boost that's okay, too. As long as you stick to the sixteen-hour Burn Zone, your body will have plenty of time to repair, replenish, and burn off fat. All that said, it takes your tummy twenty minutes to register food, so eat slowly—taking your time will help you to notice when you are sated. It also helps to eat in a tranquil setting. Stopping before you are stuffed means paying attention to the subtle shift that happens when you eat a meal. You have to "listen" for it.

What about coffee and tea during the Burn Zone? What about cream or milk?

Yes. I encourage coffee and tea—it's an appetite suppressant. Caffeine also comes with a mild diuretic effect, so drink plenty of water to compensate. Cream and milk? It's technically a cheat, but you'll be okay if you add just a splash. One tablespoon of heavy cream is better than milk. It's 50 calories, but all fat, so it shouldn't trigger insulin. If you need a little time to get used to butter or coconut oil in your beverages, go ahead. Just keep it as light as possible, and always double-check that it is sugar-free.

Can I have milk, juice, soda, sweetened coffee, or sweetened tea (iced or hot) during my Burn?

No, you can't. The one way that you can break your Cruise Control is with sugar, especially the sort that comes in beverages. Did you know that the average adult in the United States drinks an astounding 450 calories a day? Ordering a Starbucks Iced Coffee with milk? If you don't request unsweetened, a venti drink has 170 calories and 140 of those calories are sugar. Thankfully, it's also easy to cut out. So go ahead with your order, just go unsweetened and sans the milk. If you must have creamer, ask for a splash of heavy cream (yep, Starbucks has it). Better yet, stick to calorie-free drinks, and make your Cruise Control Coffee at home.

I like to work out every day. Will Cruise Control work for me?

Definitely. The fat-burning effects that come with Cruise Control are ramped up even higher when you work out. Consider that the sleek, sexy actress, dancer, model, and good friend Brooke Burke is a committed Cruiser. She exercises lots, every day, and she says that the Burn to Boost Zones give her more energy than ever before. "It used to be that I'd wake up super hungry, make a shake that probably had a thousand calories in it, do my workout, then be hungry again and have a big lunch, then I'd snack until dinnertime—I was always eating," says Brooke. "I was fit, but I was at the edge of my ideal weight, and I had to work really hard for it." Now that Brooke follows Cruise Control, she says she's never hungry and feels free and energized to work out harder. Plus, she no longer has to try so hard to be at her ideal weight.

What if I need a snack during the Burn Zone?

Have a drink. Tea, hot or iced. Sparkling water with lime, or just a big cup of ice cold water. Your belly will be full, and the hunger will pass.

Isn't breakfast the key to weight loss? How can skipping it be healthy?

First of all, you won't be skipping breakfast. Remember that you can always enjoy a creamy, frothy, delicious Cruise Control Coffee or Tea. We know from all of the studies we've gathered that the Cruise Control Diet will help you lose weight, regardless of when you choose to Boost and Burn. Also, a lot of recent research shows that skipping breakfast actually reduces the number of overall calories a person eats in a day. That said, you're free to schedule your Boost and Burn Zones whenever you like (see "Choose Your Window," page 27). Feel free to break your Burn at 7:00 or 8:00 in the morning and end your Boost at three or four in the afternoon. If you'd rather have dinner with your family a bit later, adjust your schedule. Just choose the Boost and Burn that works best for you!

Can I have a cheat meal?

After you've completed four full weeks (twenty-eight days) on Cruise Control, you can schedule a cheat meal once every ten days. This is key for sustainability and life enjoyment. But a "cheat meal" does not mean gorging at the all-you-can-eat buffet. Aim to eat a healthy meal first, and then choose a food that you've been missing. Maybe you want to go to the Cheesecake Factory for a piece of chocolate hazelnut crunch cheese-cake. Or maybe having surf and turf with all the trimmings at your favorite steakhouse sounds more appealing—go for it. Keep your indulgences to one day every ten days, and you won't lose any of the progress you've made. More often and you'll go back to burning sugar and storing fat.

I work out early and like to have a small snack or shake before I head out. Is that okay?

You'd be breaking your Burn. The best way to achieve maximum results is to stick to the Burn Zone treats. If you feel like you need something before your morning workout, have Cruise Control Coffee or Tea.

Can I still take my usual vitamins and supplements during the Burn Zone?

You sure can. However, if you burp herbs or fish oil, get woozy, or have stomach discomfort, wait until your Boost Zone to take your vitamins and supplements.

I take medications with food. How do I do this on Cruise Control?

Certain drugs can cause side effects on an empty stomach. Ibuprofen can cause stomach distress and ulcers. Iron supplements make some people feel nauseous. Metformin, a common medicine for diabetics, can do the same and may cause diarrhea to boot. It should be fine to adjust these medicines to a time after a Boost Zone Meal. Many medications might be okay after consuming the healthy fats that are in the Burn Zone foods and drinks. If you have any concerns, discuss it with your doctor.

What if I have diabetes?

If you have diabetes or take diabetes medication, it's also important for you to talk to your doctor about the Cruise Control program. Certain diabetes medications, such as metformin, are sometimes used for other conditions, such as polycystic ovary syndrome. Check your blood sugar as directed by your doctor, and adjust your medications as recommended. Close monitoring by your physician is essential because your blood sugar will decrease, and if you take medications, you could become hypoglycemic. If you repeatedly have low blood sugar, it means that your medications need to be adjusted, not that Cruise Control isn't working. When I work with diabetic clients, I insist on close monitoring by a physician to track and anticipate blood sugar changes and medication adjustments.

Can I exercise during the Burn Zone?

See chapter 8, but yes. Many people assume that the Burn Zone will be just like fasting, and they expect that they won't have the energy for exercise or to deal with physically demanding jobs. Yes, exercise and physical activity demand extra energy from the body—but you'll have plenty of it. Your body will be primed to first burn through your glycogen, the limited sugar stored in the liver. Since there is extra demand for energy during exercise, and since glycogen is limited, it runs out faster, and your body turns to fat burning—and we all have plenty of energy in our fat stores to keep us going for days on end without food.

On Cruise Control, your muscles adapt to burning fat for energy. Athletes hit the proverbial "wall" only when they haven't been adapted to a Burn/Boost style of eating. Their bodies are relying on sugar for energy (and it's limited). However, when you are adapted to burning fat, the breakdown of fat for energy is enhanced, and you won't run into any walls. Your performance won't suffer during exercise. However, during the first week or two when you are adjusting to the change from burning sugar to burning fat, you may notice a slight reduction in your physical energy. During this time you will be teaching your body to expect to use energy from fat. Be patient—you will regain your previous energy and more.

What if I need to skip a week?

The interesting outcome among the Cruisers I've worked with is that they all tell me that they don't feel as if they are *on* a diet. So, Cruisers don't usually feel like they need to "go off" Cruise Control. However, I'm a realist, so if you need to take a few days or even a week off, try to keep it to a modified Burn of ten or even eleven hours a day. You can still maximize the Burn/Boost food lists and minimize the bad guys. If you stick with Cruise Control 80 percent of the time, you'll still get plenty of benefits. Just keep in mind that the closer you stay to an eight-to-sixteen Boost-to-Burn ratio, the better and faster your results.

I'm a vegetarian/vegan. How can I make Cruise Control work for me?

Let me be straight with you. Vegans have a harder time getting their protein needs met than vegetarians. Why? Vegetarians usually allow protein-rich foods such as eggs, cottage cheese, tofu, and Greek yogurt, while vegans stick with just the plants. That doesn't make it impossible to be a vegan on Cruise Control, it just means that you'll have to pay close attention to your macronutrients. Thanks to new plant-based protein powders, you can now get safe, delicious, and low-sugar and low-carb vegan sources of protein made from peas, pumpkin seeds, sunflower seeds, hemp seeds, artichokes, quinoa, and other grains. Sometimes the science of processed foods can churn out something beneficial. This faction of the food industry has figured out how to isolate the good protein from these different plant sources and make it into a yummy, easy protein powder. Just be sure to check the labels, and then adapt as needed. I use the protein powders made by 22 Days Nutrition because they keep the ingredients simple and real (see Resources, page 304, for more information). If you're looking for dairy substitutes, coconut and almond milk are my favorites (unsweetened, of course).

Onward! The Open Road: Week Five and Beyond

Congratulations! You've reached your final destination. So, where will you go next? The road is open for your next journey.

Whether you are reading this because you've finished the Four-Week Plan or because you're ready to plan ahead, I'm glad you're here. People who think ahead about how they will continue to improve their health are more likely to do so.

I'm confident that my Cruise Control Diet is a solution to health and forever fat-burning. But I also know that our work is never really done. That's why I keep hammering home that Cruise Control is a lifestyle, not a diet. To make sustainable, long-lasting changes means making a long-term commitment. You're here because you're ready to take the steps you need to solidify your new lifestyle, to lose the rest of the weight, to maintain a healthy weight, to keep on burning fat, and to stay fit and healthy forever.

YOUR CHOICES

Whether you're already Cruising down the road and enjoying the plan just as it is, or if you're preparing to start a brand-new journey, or if you've reached your goal weight, here are some ideas of how you might like to continue on the Cruise Control lifestyle. And, whatever you choose to do, I hope that you join the thousands of other Cruisers and share your story and your success at Facebook.com/JorgeCruise. You can also help cheer other Cruisers on in their quest for better health and a thriving life. Here are some choices for you to make next.

Let Me Be Your Coach: If you are busy or looking for more variety without having to develop and create them, you can get more menus and recipes at my website, JorgeCruise.com, and have me do all the work for you with my online Platinum program. I'll provide you with new menus each week, so you never have repetitive meals, and you'll always have access to easy-to-make, delicious foods that follow Cruise Control. Studies have shown that when people are coached, they are able to lose three times more weight. That is the main reason I have developed an online resource where I can be your coach and give you new meals and meal planners that will take the stress out of weight control. If you are serious about making the change, I invite you to see what my online Platinum program has to offer at JorgeCruise.com. If this is the option that fits your lifestyle, I look forward to working with you. Learn more at platinum.jorgecruise.com.

Let the Book Coach You: You can also simply return to the first four weeks and follow the menus again. For some, there is great power in simplicity. If you enjoy a very structured routine, you may find that knowing what to eat each week from the guidelines in this book is exactly the fit for your lifestyle. If you love to cook and experiment with new foods, dive in and have fun with all the delicious recipes.

You Be the Coach: You can take your new knowledge to the next level and start making your own menus from the food lists located on page 127 or by simply reordering the meal plan as you see fit. If you love the Lemon Chicken Kale Salad (from week one, day one, page 93) feel free to have it all week long. If you want to make extra Turmeric Shrimp Fajitas (from week one, day three, page 95) and take the leftovers for lunch tomorrow, go for it! You can switch and swap any meal or snack for another meal or snack.

Cruise Control gives you the most powerful solution to gain control over your body weight, health, and wellness. It's the simplest and most effective weight-loss design that helps you gain control over cravings, changes your relationship with food, and turns your body into a fat-burning machine. Finally, here you have a method that empowers you and puts you in the driver's seat of your health. There is no more caving in, there's no more feeling guilty, there's no more feeling hopeless. This is a weight-loss lifestyle that gives you the power to be the healthiest you can be. Again, I encourage you to join the community of millions of Cruisers at Facebook.com/JorgeCruise and stay connected with me on social media and with other like-minded Cruisers to keep you *and them* on track to a healthy life (look for #CruiseControlDiet).

Safe travels to you in all of your future adventures. I know they'll be epic!

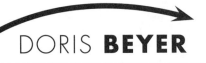

DORIS **BEYER**

AGE: 35 | WEIGHT LOST: 29 POUNDS

What everyone needs to know: I succeeded because I learned to shut down the negative voices in my head. I didn't have any faith when I started Cruise Control. I'd been trying for four long years to lose weight, and all I'd been doing was gaining more, but I knew I'd better work something out for my health. So, when I read about Jorge's plan, I thought, "What the heck. The only thing I have to lose is weight."

The eating plan was simple, and I didn't get hungry. So I started to tell myself, "Let me see what happens if I don't give up." I got online, joined in with other Cruisers, and Jorge and others gave me so many motivational tips and support that I never felt alone. I'm so glad I didn't give up, and I really did lose—the weight.

APPENDIX A

THE GROUNDBREAKING SCIENCE BEHIND CRUISE CONTROL

I t's hard to overemphasize the power of Cruise Control.

I'm seeing tremendous transformations firsthand in my clients that I've never witnessed before. I know that my past books have had great results because I've always stuck to the same formula—simple lifestyle designs based on solid scientific research. It's no different with *The Cruise Control Diet*. By building on my past recommendations for eating and moving in a way that honors how the human body is biologically designed, *The Cruise Control Diet* now brings all of your trillions of cells into perfect synchronicity for foolproof, long-lasting weight loss, fat burning, and improved health and wellness. Not only will you shed excess weight, but you'll also gain sleek, lean muscles and lose the flab. You'll have more energy each day, and you'll sleep better at night. But there's more! I've been working with thousands of people who are following Cruise Control, and I'm seeing many of them who are being told to reduce or stop the medications they were previously prescribed for high blood pressure, high cholesterol, diabetes, and heart disease. You may even recover from cancer treatment faster and more successfully. I know these are big claims—but that's the reality of what I'm seeing.

Once again, let me be clear: This is not another restrictive diet, and it's not a complicated regimen. This is a simple design for living that *is* backed by a wealth of substantial evidence. So much, in fact, that I wanted to bring it to your attention all in one place. And so, here we go.

PUMPING UP YOUR POWERHOUSES, YOUR MITOCHONDRIA

Inside all of our cells there are battery-like organelles (mini organs) called mitochondria. These mitochondria are responsible for several critical functions that keep your body healthy and young, including regulating the energy flow of your cells, promoting new cell growth, and "retiring" old and worn-out cells in your body. This is how you fight aging! These tiny organelles are behind your body's repair system. When you follow the Burn to Boost Zones each day, you'll power up your body's fat-burning mechanism by resetting your insulin levels so you'll burn more body fat for energy than sugar. The process of eating on Cruise Control powers up your mitochondria, which then improves your insulin sensitivity.

Mitochondria create most of your body's chemical energy—called adenosine triphosphate (ATP)—from the food you eat. But the key thing you need to know about mitochondria is that while they create energy (good news), they also produce waste (like a car engine produces exhaust—not so good). We call our mitochondria waste "free radicals," which are highly reactive uncharged molecules that cause many of the results we see with aging (wrinkles, aches and pains, sagging skin). A reasonable amount of this waste is expected by your body and can be routinely eliminated, but if you have too many of these troublemakers they can wreak havoc, causing aging, disease, and illness. Free radicals have been linked to cardiovascular disease, cancer, diabetes, Alzheimer's, wrinkles, sagging skin, and more.

Figuring out ways to charge up mitochondria while reducing free radicals has become the hot news in antiaging science. One company called Pulse Centers sells a machine that acts like jumper cables for your cells by using pulsed electromagnetic fields (PEMF) technology. The promise of this is that the charges improve your body's energy production, increase oxygenation, enhance circulation, promote hydration, facilitate detoxification, and help your body to absorb nutrients better. This therapy is noninvasive, noncontact, and non-pharmacological, and more than two thousand double-blind studies suggest that PEMF therapy is a safe and effective treatment and promotes and maintains general cellular health and function. But Pulse Centers are still hard to find in the United States. So, what's the less *Star Trek*-y solution to controlling free radicals? Antioxidants. Antioxidants fight free radicals. Again, your body makes its own antioxidants, but not necessarily enough to defeat these spasmodic oxygen molecules (this is one of the reasons you hear so much about getting antioxidants from certain foods or taking supplements). What your body really needs is to eat in a way that synchronizes your eating so that your body can produce its own internal antioxidants. You need to give your body time to build up these antioxidants and to burn off the toxins, which is exactly what Cruise Control does.

GIVING THE *CREW* TIME TO CLEAN AND REPAIR

Cruise Control will automatically help your body boost antioxidants and burn up free radicals by giving your cellular factories the downtime they need to clean up waste, take out the trash, and do repairs. Eating from 5:00 A.M. to midnight, like I used to, interfered with my body's maintenance time. My digestive system was so consumed with processing food that it couldn't get to its other jobs. That's why I was feeling wiped out all the time, noticing more lines on my face and fewer results from my workouts. Cutting out the foods that interfered with my body's repair crew by following the sixteen-hour Burn Zone revs up my body by giving it the time it needs to fix what gets broken each day. In addition, it also does what every cleanup crew does—takes out the trash. Remember when the *I Love Lucy* characters Lucy and Ethel went to work on the candy-wrapping assembly line? The candy never stopped coming, and they ended up stuffing the chocolates in their mouths and down their blouses. Hilarious, but seriously, this is what it's like for your body when you don't shut down the "assembly line," that is, your digestive system.

When you turn on your Cruise Control, you'll automatically lose weight, look younger, and feel healthier and happier because your Burn Zone *is* your built-in maintenance time. You can think of this as similar to the scheduled oil changes and tune-ups you make for your car. I drive a lot. If I just drove all the time, and never took a break to have my oil and other fluids changed and my engine cleaned and maintained, my car wouldn't last long. That's what your Burn Zone does. When you follow the Cruise Control eating/fasting (Boost/Burn) schedule, you give your body the time it needs to break down the food you ate. You make more energy, burn more fat, get rid of waste, and store less fat on your body.

Another way to think about this is that your body can't *take in, process, store, or absorb* energy (Boosting) while it is *cleaning up and repairing* (Burning) the aftermath of the digestive process at the same time. Did you get that? It's as if your body only has room for one set of workers. The day shift (your eight-hour Boost Zone) needs to be focused on filling your body with fuel and digesting and processing that fuel, while the night shift needs to concentrate on cleaning, restocking, repairing, and preparing *the shop* (you) for the next day shift. Your Burn Zone is the shift when cleanup, repair, and preparation happens. Back to the car analogy? You can't burn gas and fix or clean the engine at the same time. With Cruise Control you make it all automatic.

BURN OFF BELLY FAT LIKE NEVER BEFORE

Cruise Control directly burns belly fat! I've seen this firsthand with my own results and in those of thousands of clients and online Cruisers. In 2007, the *American Journal of Clinical Nutrition* published findings on two groups of subjects that both were provided the same number of calories per day, but one group had to eat within a restricted time frame (similar to the eight-hour Boost Zone). The time-restricted eaters lowered belly fat, but the anytime eaters didn't.

When you are in the Burn Zone phase of Cruise Control, your body has to work to find energy—this is part of the reason that you burn fat during the Burn Zone. People who eat all the time give their bodies constant energy (usually sugars in the form of carbohydrates) to use, so their bodies never need to access and use their body fat. Result: All-time eaters retain, and probably gain, fat. The other reason you burn off more fat is that restricting the time in which you eat your food (your Boost Zone) makes your body's metabolism shift to a higher gear—that means that your engine gets a turbo boost and burns more calories! Folks who graze all day have metabolisms that grow lazy because they never have to search for energy. Think of time-restricted eating, your eight-hour Boost Zone, as an exercise session for the inside of your body! During your sixteen-hour Burn Zone, your body will be busy burning up fat, flab, and loose skin.

One of my good friends is Dr. Daryl Gioffre, a nutritionist and longevity expert, and author of *Get Off Your Acid*. He tells me that when you do a sixteen-hour Burn Zone, you lower your blood sugar and insulin and increase your production of growth hormone (which improves your inside cellular repair crew). Gioffre explains that this fasting period increases your metabolic rate and signals your body to burn stored fat for energy. "Your body was designed to run on fat for fuel," Gioffre told me. "That's why 95 percent of calories stored on your body are stored as fat, and only 5 percent of stored energy is stored as sugar."

The Burn Zone also activates the receptors in your body that increase fat burning, while slowing cellular receptors that put the brakes on fat burning. A 2011 study of women who followed either a Cruise Control–like eating plan or a non-time-restricted plan found that the Cruisers lost more body weight and shrank their waist circumference more than those who were non-time-restricted. Cruise Control re-creates what our ancestors used to experience in times of feasts and famines—fat burning and removal of toxic waste on your body. "You're increasing human growth hormone, so your body goes into a state of autophagy," says Gioffre. Autophagy is your body's cellular recycling program because it causes the breakdown of cellular waste and the building of new and better cells. As he further explains, "Autophagy bumps your body into a high metabolic state because it has to work hard to remove and recycle cellular debris." That means that you burn more calories and fat overall, especially belly fat. This concept was echoed by health expert Naomi Whittel, author of the popular book *Glow 15*. As she put it to me: "Our bodies have trillions of cells, and each one comes with a mechanism that eats up the waste, removes the debris, and replaces any damaged parts of the cells so that we can have more energy and vitality, and so we can look younger. This process is autophagy."

BECOME A DISEASE-FIGHTING MACHINE

It's great to look great, but I'm just getting started on the health benefits you'll receive from this simple lifestyle plan. Studies show that eating on Cruise Control will lower your risk of heart disease, diabetes, and cancer. Many of my Cruising clients have already started telling me about these miracles. Let's take a look.

Beat Heart Disease

Most cases of heart disease are caused by fat deposits on your arterial walls, the tubes that carry blood from your heart. Excess fat in your body causes inflammation, including inflammation in your arteries.

Cruise Control to the rescue! When you follow the Cruise Control Boost/Burn schedule, you will naturally prepare your body to burn more fat and to store less. When you do this, you reduce fat in the body, and that decreases inflammation. When you diminish fatty deposits, it suggests that they aren't floating around your arteries, or stuck to the walls of your arteries as fatty plaque. When you clear out your tubes, you lessen your chance of blockage to the heart—and that decreases your heart disease risk. How much? According to a 2011 study, you can have a 58 percent lower risk of heart disease when you commit to a scheduled fast or, better yet, a sixteen-hour Burn Zone. The study was presented at the 2011 conference of the American College of Cardiology, and the researchers found no changes in heart disease risk among the people who didn't have a regular fasting plan. Other studies have found similar evidence.

I'm seeing dramatic results in my Cruising clients. One client named Stan recently told me that his doctor's jaw dropped at a recent visit when his once dangerously high blood pressure had plummeted to an entirely safe range and he lost ninety pounds. And Dolly, another Cruise Control devotee, told me that her blood pressure is now healthy and she's improved her heart health.

Slash Your Diabetes Risk

More than 30 million Americans have diabetes, 84 million have prediabetes, and every year 1.5 million new cases of diabetes are identified. It's a serious problem. There are two types of diabetes. Type 1 diabetes is a condition—usually diagnosed in children (once upon a time it was called childhood diabetes)—where the body cannot produce insulin. This happens when a person's immune system attacks the pancreas cells that make insulin.

Type 2 diabetes is caused by excessively and chronically high sugar in the blood. This high sugar creates an overwhelming demand on your pancreas to produce insulin. At first, your pancreas keeps up with the excess sugar by producing more insulin, but over time it can't keep up. Remember, insulin is the hormone that makes decisions about what is to be done with your blood sugar and how it needs to be stored, and when it gets put away, it gets put away as fat. When you get too much sugar (and the vast majority of us do because all carbohydrates are really just various forms of sugar), your pancreas fizzles out, and your body also becomes increasingly resistant to the insulin that is produced (called insulin resistance). A type 2 diabetic basically has a sugar-addicted and sugar-dependent body. After years of overworking the system, your body eventually begins to lose the ability to react appropriately to the insulin—what I explained earlier to be insulin resistance. Having type 2 diabetes doesn't just mean that you carry around a bunch of extra weight and you get high blood sugar readings at the doctor (although you will). Without lifestyle changes it often causes blindness, amputation of limbs, and early death.

Diabetes is another case where you need to give your body time in both the Boost (eating foods that boost insulin resistance) and the Burn (not eating insulin-triggering foods) Zones to get your body back to peak performance. How does this work? According to leading circadian rhythm expert Dr. Satchin Panda from the Salk Institute, it turns out that your pancreas has its own clock, which tells it to inhibit the production of insulin at night. Also, your brain's clock releases increased amounts of the sleep hormone melatonin at night, and melatonin also tells your pancreas to suppress insulin production. If you eat late into the night while your pancreas is resting and repairing, it won't release the insulin necessary to handle and regulate your blood sugar. This continues the defeating cycle of insulin resistance, high blood sugar, and increased diabetes risk. All that stops when you harness your eating with Burn and Boost Zones because you respect your entire body's biological needs for rest and repair. This helps bring back pancreatic performance, lowers blood sugar, and increases insulin resistance.

In other words, as Dr. Jason Fung, author of *The Complete Guide to Fasting*, explains, type 2 diabetes is "an entirely reversible disease with weight loss. The essence of the disease is really that there is too much sugar in the body. All you need to do is eliminate the sugar in your body." That's what Cruise Control does. My Cruising clients Laura and Jolene were both able to dramatically lower their diabetes medications and their blood sugar levels by following the sixteen-hour Burn and the eight-hour Boost Zones for just two weeks.

Destroy Cancer

Cancer is a blanket name given to a group of related diseases that can occur in just about every area in the body.

Healthy cells in your body have a certain life span—they are supposed to die, divide, or be replaced at a certain time. Your cells age just like you age. Cancer cells crowd out healthy cells, and cancer can spread from one area to another (called metastasis). Cancer is always called by where it started. So if you are diagnosed with lung cancer, even if it spreads (or metastasizes) to your bones, it is still referred to as lung cancer.

Some tumors grow slowly; others grow and spread fast. Different treatments work for different types of cancers, but one thing that lowers the risk of all cancers *and* improves the treatment and outcome if you *do* have cancer is adopting a firm Boost and Burn Zone.

When you eat morning, noon, and night, you are putting constant demands on your body. That's the big problem. The average person eats from five to ten times a day over a fifteen-hour period. Where's the downtime? When you follow the Boost/Burn schedule, you are creating the needed downtime, and you'll ramp up your immune system by honoring your body's biological rhythm. The sixteen-hour Burn Zone gives your brain and your body the time it needs to rest and repair. If you are eating from dawn to dusk, your immune system is weakened. When that happens, your immune system's ability to find cancerous cells stops working. But if you are on Cruise Control, you'll give your body the power to fight off cancer successfully.

SHARPEN YOUR MIND

For all the physical promise of going on Cruise Control, one of the things I love best is that following a Boost/Burn Zone schedule on a daily basis recharges your brain in a manner that will turn back the clock on your memory, clarity, and focus. Plus, you will reduce stress, anxiety, and depression and have a stronger and more stable emotional balance than ever before. In my view—and pun intended—nourishing and fortifying your mind on Cruise Control is a *no-brainer.*

Let me break it down for you: Just about every part of your brain has its own clock or twenty-four-hour rhythmic cycle that it flows to, and if these brain clocks aren't functioning or "keeping time" correctly, you will be vulnerable to all sorts of mind mayhem. Cruise Control resets your mind clocks by helping you to automate the creation of newer, better brain cells and amplified neural connections (that means you'll be smarter). How does this work?

It's back to the Boost/Burn Zone. When you incorporate the sixteen-hour Burn Zone on a regular schedule, your brain starts producing higher amounts of a miracle brain protein called brain-derived neurotrophic factor (BDNF), which helps to grow sparkling new stem cells in your brain. Stem cells are the cells that start out in an embryo and have the magical power of morphing into whatever sort of cell you might need. That means they can replace damaged cells with new healthy ones. You may have heard some of the antiaging properties of stem cells. Well, listen up. Until relatively recently, we thought that stem cells were for kids and that once you were grown, you didn't make stem cells. Now we know that, thanks to BDNF, your brain can still produce new stem cells that pump up your remembering abilities and your capacity to learn new things. All you have to do to encourage this brain regeneration is to turn on Cruise Control.

The stem-cell boosting protein also strengthens your synapses (the place where your nerve cells pass messages and directions to one another), which indicates that the only thing you're going to *forget* about is having memory lapses or airhead moments—because they won't be happening. Finally, having a regular Burn Zone time gives your brain the freedom to repair and renew all parts of your gray matter, including the increase of your own production of antioxidants. The alternative, eating from 5:00 A.M. to midnight, never gives your brain a chance to do anything but deal with the processing of incoming energy.

The other way that you can promote peak brain power is by eating less overall, and by letting yourself *get* hungry. Probably the most well-known day for overeating is Thanksgiving. We are all familiar with the food coma we feel after turkey with all the trimmings. That enormous feast takes a massive toll on your body. You feel sluggish because all of your internal factories have been called upon to process those thousands of calories. Sending nutrients to your brain is not the priority. That's why the most popular activity on T-day is to *watch* football, not to *play* it. With all of your blood going to your digestive system, less blood is available to go to your muscles or your lungs. Cruise Control clients

Renee, Cathy, Angela, Leslie, and Rochelle (to name just a few) all tell me that they have more energy and incredible mindfulness compared to their old all-day-long eating habits.

Finally, keeping your insulin levels low also boosts your memory. Turns out that the higher your insulin levels, the less able you'll be to retain memories. On the flip side, keep insulin low, and your mental recall seems to improve. That's what you'll do on Cruise Control.

LIVE A LONGER, HEALTHIER LIFE

Cruise Control taps into powerful natural healing and regenerative processes in your brain and body that can help you to live longer and better. When you buy a new car, everything works great. But after a few years, it starts to get a little beat up and needs more maintenance. You need to replace the brake pads, then the battery, then more and more parts. Eventually, the car is breaking down all the time and costing thousands of dollars to maintain. Does it make sense to keep it around? Likely not. So you get rid of it and buy a snazzy new car. You can't do this with your body. You get one machine that is to last your lifetime—so our focus must be on how to maintain and care for our bodies and brains to help them to age slowly and to perform better for longer.

Eating on a regular Boost to Burn schedule has been scientifically shown to reduce most age-related conditions and diseases and to help you to live healthier and happier into your later years. How this works is multifaceted, involving several different hormonal reactions, neural impulses, mitochondrial functioning, cell repair, and more. Researchers are still uncovering all of the ways that being on Cruise Control drives you to live longer, but here's a sampling of some of the most promising age-defying benefits that you'll get from following a regular Boost to Burn cycle:

- Consistently lowering insulin levels, with improvement of overall insulin sensitivity.
- Increasing cellular activity, repair, and regeneration.
- Improving quality and quantity of sleep.
- Protecting cells from stress and toxic damage.

- Enhancing neural connections in your brain.
- Keeping mitochondria (your cell powerhouses) plentiful and productive.
- Ramping up cellular waste removal and recycling.
- Decreasing chronic inflammation.
- Recharging your immune system.
- Creating new stem cells.

One of the ways that your body naturally does all this is with a confusingly named hormone called human growth hormone. As the name implies, human growth hormone plays a critical role in the growing and developing bodies of children and adolescents, but this hormone also plays a core part in the repair processes that happen in all human bodies each night by telling certain cells to divide and regenerate. A lot of my female clients don't like the sound of this hormone because they equate it with *growing* bigger muscles, but that's not how growth hormone works. Human growth hormone is all about encouraging your cells to duplicate, repair, and regenerate.

Growth hormone peaks during puberty and then gradually decreases with age. Figuring out how to keep this antiaging hormone from diminishing can help your body stay young, and the best way to do this is to have strong and synchronized clocks in your body. That's great news because harmonizing your clocks is something that is built right into the Cruise Control design.

Deficient growth hormone levels in adults lead to more body fat, less muscle mass, and weak bones. Each night when you sleep, growth hormone is released, and it peaks just before waking, at 4:00 A.M. or so. Why can't we just take growth hormone in a pill? You can, but the results are mixed.

One study found that after six months of taking a growth hormone supplement, subjects lost 5.3 pounds of fat while increasing bone and muscle mass by 8.2 pounds. Remember, muscle is much leaner than fat, so gaining muscle doesn't mean you look bigger or have hulking muscles—it means that you look slim and sleek. However, growth hormone that isn't made naturally comes with side effects that include dangerously elevated blood sugar, blood pressure, and some indication that cancer and heart disease risk increase. Thankfully, Cruise Control taps your body's cellular system to create natural growth hormone. How? It's back to the Burn and Boost Zones. The most potent way to signal growth hormone is to *not* eat for sixteen hours, but remember, you'll be fasting with fat, so you'll never feel like you're starving, but you'll preserve all the benefits of fasting. Studies show that following this method can double your production of growth hormone in just five days!

APPENDIX B

RESOURCES

always love the resource section of books. It's where you get to pick the author's brain and get all sorts of extra ideas, tools, and tips. That's what I've tried to do here. On the next few pages, you'll find the websites, cookbooks, health and wellness books, products, apps, podcasts, experts, and institutes that I recommend. The people I've included here are those with whom I've developed a close personal and professional relationship. That's not saying that everything you find here in the Resources will be 100 percent in agreement with Cruise Control, but you can trust these resources to honestly tell you whether or not they are compliant with the Cruiser lifestyle. Just rely on this book, my website, and my social media pages as your primary go-to resources and toolbox. You may also have products and people you value that aren't included on this list. Just use your own best judgment, and when it comes to products, always do your homework. Read the fine print, the ingredients, and the nutrient information. And always use the wide-reaching Internet with intelligence and caution. 'Nuff said.

WEBSITES

Jorge Cruise: jorgecruise.com
Welcome to my home on the World Wide Web. This is where you'll take your learning to a new level with Cruise Control Platinum. This exclusive coaching opportunity is geared to upgrade your nutrition, fitness, recovery, and mindset. My mission is to give you intimate coaching that

will help you automate your life. My clients get direct access via live support in addition to events three times per year.

Platinum.jorgecruise.com
Facebook: facebook.com/jorgecruise
Instagram: @jorgecruise
Twitter: @jorgecruise

Dr. Weil: drweil.com

Dr. Andrew Weil is an integrative medical practitioner and teacher of all things health and wellness. I especially like his website for the incredible diet, supplement, and nutrition information available.

Brooke Burke: brookeburke.com

I have to plug Brooke, of course, but not just because she's one of my best friends. You'll find great fitness routines and exercise videos on Brooke's site that are a perfect addition to the Cruise Control Workouts.

Intensive Dietary Management: idmprogram.com

Dr. Jason Fung is the medical director at Intensive Dietary Management (IDM) program and author of *The Complete Guide to Intermittent Fasting*. The IDM program offers support and education to help with weight loss, reverse type 2 diabetes, and more.

The Primal Blueprint: primalblueprint.com

Mark Sisson, the founder of Primal Blueprint, has set up his website with educational courses, a podcast, helpful tips, and approved products. Many of Sisson's books offer recipes and eating tips that are Cruise Control–friendly and delicious.

Naomi Whittel: naomiwhittel.com

Self-described wellness explorer Naomi Whittel, author of *Glow15*, offers recipes, products, and strategies based on the Nobel Prize science on autophagy (your body's ability to discard and recycle cellular waste) and how it affects your aging and your health. Whittel applies the science available to provide practical and simple solutions for improving your health and reducing the signs of aging with nutrition, exercise, sleep, and stress reduction. You'll find simple-to-follow ideas for looking and feeling your best, as well as natural products that support your body's ability to recycle, repair, and replenish itself.

COOKBOOKS

Cruise Control gives you more than fifty-five recipes and four weeks of meal plans that will keep you and your family satisfied and healthy for a long time. You can feel safe and secure knowing that this is the one place you can come to when you want to stick to the fully Cruise Control–approved foods. That said, I love cookbooks! I like looking at color pictures of delicious-looking meals, and I'm always on the hunt for something new to try. Plus, there are many cookbooks out there that include, enhance, and inspire Cruise Control–friendly recipes. You might have to make a switch here or there, but that's how new and delicious meals are born (don't forget to share them with other Cruisers at facebook.com/jorgecruise). Experiment and enjoy the great abundance we are blessed to have available. Here are some of my favorites.

Fast Food, Good Food
BY ANDREW WEIL, M.D.
Dr. Weil likes to cook, but he isn't crazy about complicated or time-consuming recipes or hard-to-find ingredients. His focus is on the freshest ingredients of the best quality for your health, and he wants you to have fun. Here you can find more than 150 of Dr. Weil's own favorite fast recipes for soups, salads, main courses, and more. Learn how to prepare healthy and delicious foods that will lower inflammation and improve your health but won't stress you out in the process.

True Food: Seasonal, Sustainable, Simple, Pure
BY ANDREW WEIL, M.D., AND SAM FOX
Dr. Weil collaborated with coauthor Sam Fox, a third-generation restaurateur and highly skilled chef, to design, create, and ultimately open the first True Food Kitchen restaurant in Phoenix in 2008. True Food Kitchen restaurants are based on the philosophy that food can be delicious, nutritious, and conscious. This book is a generous sampling of Dr.

Weil's restaurant in print. You'll find more than 125 recipes for fresh, flavorful, and healthy dishes that always prioritize fresh, local, organic, and in-season ingredients.

The Keto Reset Diet

BY MARK SISSON

The world-renowned proponent of the benefits of living the hunter-gatherer lifestyle is back. Here, Sisson shares more scientific developments and information that offer additional support for keto-adapting your body. You'll learn why our ancestors still hold the key to the best way to reverse aging, increase energy, and improve health and happiness. My friend Sisson details how modeling the nomad's lifestyle of those who lived thousands of years before us is the single most powerful way to decrease inflammation, aging, and disease and to create peak performance. Sisson guides you, step-by-step, on how to reprogram your body to burn fat at a sensible pace. You'll find a twenty-one-day meal plan and more than one hundred recipes to make going keto enjoyable and delicious while rebooting your system for better health without the burnout that can come from other keto plans.

The Keto Reset Diet Cookbook

BY MARK SISSON AND BRAD KEARNS

This is the perfect addition to Sisson's Keto Reset Diet. Mark Sisson, of the Primal Kitchen, and coauthor Brad Kearns bring you 150 low-carb, high-fat ketogenic recipes. Here you'll find many options that are Cruise Control–friendly and will keep you burning fat.

Fuel Up

BY LAIRD HAMILTON

Surfer Laird Hamilton brings you his take on healthy and exotic recipes for high performance that he's collected from his world travels. Hamilton's recipes highlight "plants and animals," as well as extra-virgin olive oil, avocado oil, and macadamia nuts. Yup, Hamilton has embraced healthy fats just like Cruise Control. So, you'll find plenty of yummy additions that incorporate flavors from all over the globe to add to your Cruise Control eating.

The Oz Family Kitchen
BY LISA OZ AND MEHMET OZ, M.D.

The Ozes focus on family-friendly recipes and their book, *The Oz Family Kitchen,* includes more than one hundred simple, delicious, real-food recipes. So don't just expect to find kale and an occasional walnut. The Ozes have four kids, and they say the key to eating healthily as a family is all in the planning and, of course, making meals your kids will actually eat. So, you'll find great strategies here for getting organized for healthy foods your whole clan will love.

The Plant Paradox Cookbook
BY DR. STEVEN R. GUNDRY, M.D.

Here you'll find one hundred recipes that help you lose weight and are focused on healing your gut and living lectin-free. Dr. Gundry does a great job of teaching you how to avoid hidden toxins in your foods that can harm your digestive system and cause widespread inflammation, weight gain, and illness. This cookbook also comes with some great kitchen hacks to save you time while still serving up delicious meals.

HEALTH & WELLNESS RESOURCES (BOOKS)

I'll never stop learning, investigating, and keeping my mind open to new and various health and wellness ideas—and neither should you. Here are the books by health and wellness experts who have inspired my journey.

Mind Over Meds
BY ANDREW WEIL, M.D.

This book educates you on how our society has become overreliant on medications to solve our problems, and how, in many cases, they hurt your health instead of healing you. Dr. Weil teaches you to know when drugs are necessary, when alternatives might be better, and when to let your body heal on its own.

The Obesity Code: Unlocking the Secrets of Weight Loss
BY DR. JASON FUNG, M.D.

Dr. Fung takes you into the science of how your body's own insulin is the key to controlling your weight, how most of us get it wrong, and how, when, and what to eat to get to your forever healthy weight. Dr. Fung shares essential information for cracking the obesity epidemic.

The Complete Guide to Fasting
BY DR. JASON FUNG, M.D., AND JIMMY MOORE
This book was a vital part of the development of Cruise Control. Dr. Fung and his coauthor, Jimmy Moore, deconstruct the concept of fasting, from ancient to modern strategies, into entirely understandable chunks that make it easy to see why fasting works so powerfully on the body. This book will teach you how to heal your body with regular, intermittent, alternate-day, and extended fasting.

Own the Day, Own Your Life
BY AUBREY MARCUS
Do you dare to be changed in just one day? I love this book for how Marcus brings home the empowering message of what can be done in that twenty-four-hour period that we all live in each day. I get tingles when I read just a single page of this book! Marcus has an exhilarating way of presenting information for optimizing your life by examining one day—this day!—and then learning to extend your coming days to live a more conscious life in your daily living, working, learning, eating, training, playing, sleeping, and sex.

Awaken the Giant Within
BY TONY ROBBINS
Tony was one of the first people in my life who woke me up and inspired me to the fact that I could take charge of my own life and make it exactly what I wanted. That was more than twenty years ago. I was lucky enough to work with Tony back when his powerful enthusiasm was just beginning to catch the world on fire. Tony is a master of motivation, and his use of psychological strategies to enhance personal achievement is unparalleled. If you've never read this classic, get it. It's something that should be on every bookshelf.

Get Off Your Acid
BY DR. DARYL GIOFFRE, M.D.
Dr. Gioffre is a longevity, health, and wellness expert and chiropractor in New York. His passion is teaching people how to live balanced lives

for peak performance and optimal health. Most of us eat diets that chronically exacerbate a level of acidity that hurts our guts, causes system-wide inflammation and disease, and accelerates aging. Dr. Gioffre teaches you how to balance out the microbiome in your digestive tract to get on track to good health in just seven days. This book is informative and easy to read. It contains approachable and tasty recipes that show you how to introduce more alkaline-friendly foods and reduce acidic ones for better balance and health.

Food Can Fix It
BY DR. MEHMET OZ, M.D.

Dr. Oz shares his latest take on using superfoods that fight fat, turn back the clock on aging, and boost your health overall. Many of his favorite foods and recipes overlap with the Cruise Control way of life. Dr. Oz also includes a nice breakdown of food fixes for different issues, including pain, fatigue, heart health, a healthy gut, skin, hair, and more.

The 6 Keys: Unlock Your Genetic Potential for Ageless Strength, Health, and Beauty
BY JILLIAN MICHAELS

Unlock the potential that already exists inside all your trillions of cells. Jillian takes us through the steps to live better, longer. Why do some people die two weeks into retirement while others are still driving to the store in their nineties? Jillian takes a microscopic approach into antiaging and puts the power of staying young in your hands. She gives you permission to care about your appearance, sex life, and energy. Her message is one of longevity with vitality, immunity, and vigor—and how to look hot and to have it all. You can take action to reverse aging, amplify health and beauty, and reach optimal health—Jillian says so.

The Circadian Code
BY SATCHIN PANDA, PH.D.

If there's one expert who knows how the body's rhythm works, it's Dr. Panda. His lab at the Salk Institute is dedicated to studying how the trillions of timekeepers inside your cells are influenced by diet, activity, sleep, and more. His book details the science in easy-to-understand language that explains how you can change your body's clock to lose weight, increase energy, and transform your health.

Glow15: A Science-Based Plan to Lose Weight, Revitalize Your Skin, and Invigorate Your Life

BY NAOMI WHITTEL

This is the story of one powerful woman and her journey to transform the health of millions. Learn how to shift your eating and activity patterns to harness your body's ability to remove toxic waste and to recycle cells for better health. Naomi has found a nutritional strategy to power your cells and help your body to recycle, repair, and rejuvenate. Follow Naomi's advice, and you'll improve your energy and health, have more luxuriant hair and skin, and be more fit and slim. You'll find a simple-to-follow plan for looking and feeling your best.

Deep Nutrition: Why Your Genes Need Traditional Food

BY CATE SHANAHAN, M.D.

Dr. Shanahan has a brilliant mind and takes the care and time to dissect and explain every nuance of nutrition and how our modern eating habits sabotage our health. This book is exquisitely researched and thoroughly covers all of the latest nutrition science. Dr. Shanahan details strategies for how to get back to our roots and eat like our ancestors to reduce illness, inflammation, and disease, and to achieve optimal health and well-being.

CRUISE CONTROL–APPROVED PRODUCTS

My team and I have personally tested all of the following products, and I love them. If I didn't, you wouldn't find them here. If you see our Cruise Control seal, you'll know that these products can be used in either the Burn or Boost Zone and some can be used in both. In addition, I've also received positive reviews from thousands of clients on these products. All of this lets you know that I've personally vetted these items for Cruise Control. I have a personal relationship with each of these Cruise Control–approved companies, and I highly recommend and support not only their products but their core values and mission.

On-the-Go Snacks

These are my favorite snacks to carry with me just about anywhere I go. I do always first recommend making fresh Cruise Control foods whenever possible, but when you can't be at home, these foods can really come in handy. Many are available in health food and specialty grocery stores, and all are available online.

FBOMB NUT BUTTERS & OILS

dropanfbomb.com

I almost always have some of these packets in my bag. FBOMBs (*F* as in "fat") are natural grab-and-go sources of healthy fats and nut butters. These single-serve packets come in a variety that includes MCT oil and coconut oil, macadamia nut butter with sea salt. Other combinations include blends of coconut oil, pecan, or chocolate flavors. These make great accompaniments for backpackers, cyclists, and other outdoor enthusiasts. The packets are all approved for your Burn Zone and are great dropped in a cup of coffee or tea, or used as a salad dressing with a squeeze of fresh lemon or lime at any meal.

CHOMPS

chomps.com

These are the healthy version of those jerky sticks that you see at the quick stop markets. Made with 100 percent grass-fed and grass-finished beef, venison, and free-range antibiotic-free turkey, Chomps are also gluten, GMO, hormone, and sugar free. I love Chomps' ingredient list. Unlike most fast-food snacks, you can pronounce and define each ingredient included without searching online.

PARM CRISPS

parmcrisps.com

I'll warn you right up front. These are addictive! These little crisps, made with 100 percent aged Parmesan cheese, are great for snacking, but that's not all. I love to crumble and sprinkle them on top of just about any soup or salad. These are gluten-free and come with zero carbs; the same *cannot* be said for carb-laden croutons.

DNX BARS

dnxbar.com

Here's another great way to get your protein while on the go. DNX Bars are made with 100 percent grass-fed beef, bison, and free-range chicken and are combined with a variety of fruits, vegetables, and spices. They have no added sugar, sodium, artificial ingredients, or preservatives. The protein used is free of hormones and antibiotics (safe for you and your kids). These can be used as a Boost Zone replacement snack or small meal.

22 DAYS NUTRITION PROTEIN POWDERS

22daysnutrition.com

Here you'll find organic protein powders and bars that are always plant-based, organic, gluten-free, non-GMO, and around 20 grams of protein (from pea, flax, and sacha inchi protein) per serving. I really like the taste of these powders, and I love that the ingredients are so consciously sourced.

Treats

Many of the following treats are also easy to carry along with you to have on the road, at work, or when traveling.

KETO-SNAPS

keto-snaps.com

These crispy little cookies taste like vanilla and cinnamon. They are delicious, are Cruise Control–friendly (in the Boost Zone), and are wheat-free, gluten-free, preservative- and additive-free, and non-GMO. My whole family loves Keto-Snaps.

CRUISE CONTROL CHOCOLATE

jorgecruise.com

The following three products have helped me conquer the night. One of my dearest friends, Heath Squier, for the last 15 years has created the world's most famous low-carb products under Julian Bakery. He is truly an innovator when it comes to creating the most delicious, low-carb, healthy-fat products. I'm thrilled to share with you the three products that he formulated for Cruise Control. These are not just healthy but extremely delicious and addicting. It's how I like to end my night with my clients and my family. If you need something to satisfy your chocolate craving that won't detour your weight loss or fat burning on Cruise Control, look no further. My new chocolate bar will satisfy your sweet tooth while keeping you on the road Cruising to better health. These vegan-friendly bars are made of 75 percent rich dark chocolate and feature MCT oils. Cruise Control Chocolate bars are GMO-free and sweetened with monk fruit. You're welcome.

CRUISE CONTROL BROWNIE

jorgecruise.com

Who doesn't want to have a dessert that doesn't compromise one's waistline? I crave chocolate at night and this delicious brownie satisfies my cravings. This new brownie line is rich and chocolate flavored, and tastes just like a brownie without the carbs and added sugar. It is sweetened with monk fruit and infused with refined C8 MCT oil.

CRUISE CONTROL FAT SHAKE

jorgecruise.com

Enjoy a Cruise Control–approved chocolate shake made with coconut oil, grass-fed butter, avocado oil, collagen, and other MCT oils. This shake tastes amazing, and it helps you keep on burning fat and losing weight.

CRUISE CONTROL FAT BARS

jorgecruise.com

I've designed a Cruise Control–approved meal replacement bar that provides fat-burning MCT oils and healthy protein, and keeps your carbs low—plus, it's full of chocolatey goodness.

CRUISE CONTROL GRANOLA

jorgecruise.com

Just like many of you I like to snack, but you have to learn how to snack the right way. This line of granola is delicious on its own and can even be added to other food for a crunch. The granola is high in egg-white protein, moderate in fat, has a delicious chocolate taste, is sweetened with monk fruit and some organic seeds, and includes refined C8 MCT oil.

KILLER CREAMERY

killercreamery.com

Low-carb and keto-friendly ice cream sweetened with Cruise Control–friendly stevia and erythritol, Killer Creamery includes flavors from vanilla and chocolate to Jam Session (black raspberry) and No Judge Mint (mint chip).

FAT SNAX

fatsnax.com

This company makes Cruise Control–friendly keto and low-carb cookies and teas. Chocolate chip, peanut butter, or lemon, Fat Snax Cookies are crafted with almond flour, butter, and coconut flour and sweetened with Cruise Control–friendly sweeteners. The Fat Tea blends instantly mix into hot or cold water and are made with Japanese matcha powder and MCT oils. They are sweetened with Cruise Control–friendly stevia and xylitol.

Sweeteners

SWERVE

swervesweet.com

I love the versatility of Swerve sweetener. It's made with Cruise Control–friendly sweeteners that are zero calories and are made from natural fruits and vegetables. The coolest thing about Swerve (and the reason it is my go-to sweetener) is that it comes in all sorts of styles for any of your baking needs. You can find it granulated for baking, confectioners' style for frosting, brown sugar style, and that's not all. Swerve makes cookie, cake, and pancake mixes, too.

Broth

KETTLE & FIRE

kettleandfire.com

I fully believe in the health benefits of bone broth for protecting your joints, enhancing gut health, lowering inflammation, reducing aches and pain, and maintaining glowing skin. That said, I have no time to make a good bone broth at home. Kettle & Fire is the next best thing to homemade. Their broth is slow-simmered for ten to twenty-four hours at an ideal temperature to allow nutrients, collagen, and amino acids to soak into the broth. They have options of 100 percent grass-fed beef, organic chicken bones, and a blended mushroom and chicken broth. They also make several soups. All are Cruise Control–friendly.

Veggies
CECE'S VEGGIE CO.
cecesveggieco.com
You may have seen Cece's spiralized and riced veggies the last time you were in the produce section at your grocery store. They are popping up in several major chains and are also available online. These fresh-made packets of zucchini, butternut squash, beets, cauliflower, broccoli, and more come in spaghetti and linguine pasta shapes, and in a riced version. These are done in under fifteen minutes and have become a staple in my home.

Pasta
PALMINI
eatpalmini.com
If you want to trick your kids, spiralized beets and squash aren't going to cut it. If you have picky eaters at home, this is the pasta substitute for you. Made from healthy hearts of palm, Palmini can be made fast with a zap and tastes amazingly like real pasta.

Crusts
CALI'FLOUR FOODS
califlourfoods.com
Another incredible time-saver made from fresh ingredients. Cali'flour crusts are from cauliflower and other Cruise Control–friendly vegetables, along with almond flour, flax meal, olive oil, Himalayan pink salt, and other healthy ingredients. These are low-carb, gluten- and grain-free, and Cruise Control–friendly for making an at-home Boost Zone pizza.

Beverages
CRUISE CONTROL COFFEE
jorgecruise.com
I've already talked up my coffee (see more details in chapter 2, page 37), and that's because I believe it's a vital part of keeping you on your fat-burning, health-boosting journey. There's no other instant and healthy-fat enriched coffee on the market. These coffees will keep your energy revved and your appetite suppressed, and you'll be burning fat for longer.

ZEVIA

zevia.com

This is my go-to soda. Zevia is a line of zero-calorie sodas that are sweetened with Cruise Control–friendly stevia. They come in tons of flavors, including black cherry, cola, grape, orange, ginger ale, and many more. And don't just stop at the sodas. Zevia now has energy drinks, sparkling waters, and mixers for your cocktails. All are calorie-free and sweetened with stevia.

CRIO BRU

criobru.com

This is chocolate turned coffee. Roasted, ground, and brewed just like coffee, Crio Bru is made from 100 percent cacao beans and has the aroma of pure dark chocolate.

FAT-BURNING LEMONADE

onebodyonelife.com/shop/fat-burning-lemonade/

Sweetened with stevia and made with L-carnitine to improve energy, clear your complexion, reduce inflammation, balance pH levels, and more, these instant lemonade packets can easily be mixed in water.

STUR

sturdrinks.com

Stur's tagline is "love water naturally," which basically describes what this natural water flavor enhancer does for those water-haters out there. Stur uses real fruit and vegetable extracts and stevia sweetener to make zero-calorie water enhancers.

PIQUE TEA

piquetea.com

Coffee isn't the only cold brew in town. Pique Tea has designed a method for cold brewing and crystallizing their tea into delicious packets that are pure and potent and have up to twelve times more antioxidants compared to regular tea. This company uses premium, organic tea leaves from family-owned farms.

Alcohol

Before you get too excited, these brands still don't give you a free pass to drink with abandon or unlimited, open access to alcohol. Be smart. The limits discussed on pages 249–50 still apply. That said, I love these companies for the natural and organic ingredients and processes they use to produce beverages that are superior to their competitors.

DRY FARM WINES

dryfarmwines.com

Dry Farm Wines produces high-quality natural wines from small, sustainable family farms. Dry Farm Wines are organic, sugar-free, carb-free, and mold-free. They test each wine to guarantee that it is low in sulfites (less than 75 ppm) and do not include any additives. Their wines taste fresh and vibrant. You won't be disappointed.

CASAMIGOS TEQUILA

casamigostequila.com

Yep, this is the "George Clooney" tequila, and I do love it. This award-winning tequila is known for being made from 100 percent blue weber agave, and for slow cooking, slow fermentation, and delicious results. Casamigos Tequila is so smooth that you won't need to cover the taste with salt or lime.

Condiments

PRIMAL KITCHEN

primalkitchen.com

There are just no other better Cruise Control–friendly condiments than those made by Mark Sisson of The Primal Kitchen. Here you'll find healthy-fat condiments that are free of added sugars and carbs. If you're looking for convenience and quality, you can't go wrong with Mark's products.

Yogurt

PEAK YOGURT

peakyogurt.com

This is my go-to yogurt because it is specifically designed to be lower in sugars than other yogurts and it's also super creamy and delicious.

Creamer

CRUISE CONTROL CREAMER

jorgecruise.com

This is my Cruise Control–designed powdered creamer that you can carry with you to add to your coffee or tea. Here you'll find healthy coconut oil, grass-fed butter, and MCTs that will help keep you energized and in a fat-burning state.

LAIRD SUPERFOOD

lairdsuperfood.com

Surfer Laird Hamilton has designed some delicious "beverage enhancers" that can be added to your coffee, teas, and smoothies. Here you'll find healthy coconut oil with coconut milk powder. Available in original and in anti-inflammatory turmeric flavors.

SOURCING GOOD FOOD

DAILY HARVEST

dailyharvestmarket.com

Locally grown produce delivery services to Southern California.

MARGEAUX & LINDA'S VEGAN KITCHEN

mlvegankitchen.com

This mother, brother, and daughter team work together to bring you food that is organic, vegan, anti-inflammatory, non-GMO, and more.

SUNLIFE ORGANICS

sunlifeorganics.com

Providing organic juices and more to Southern California, SunLife Organics also provides online products, including nuts, seeds, cacao powder, and more.

FACTOR 75

factor75.com

Finally, a healthy meal company that can deliver to you in all forty-eight continental states (sorry, Alaska and Hawaii, but maybe soon). Choose your meals and sit back and relax. You can have Cruise Control meals waiting for you, fresh and ready, at the end of a long workday. Don't worry, Factor 75 has figured out a way to keep your foods safely cold until you get home.

SUPPLEMENTS

Note, these featured products are brands and supplements I like based on their ingredient list and the fact that they are all available for purchase by the general public (without going through a medical professional). However, I always recommend that you speak with your healthcare practitioner before taking any new supplements or changing supplement brands or dosage.

Electrolytes

LYTELINE

lyteline.com

Your cells need electrolytes to stay stable and to carry electrical charges required for nerve cells to communicate. I've fallen in love with the electrolyte solution these guys make called LyteShow. It's a concentrate that you can add to water, it's made without added sugars or artificial flavors or colors, and it's made with natural ingredients. I love the taste, and a little goes a long way. I like to use these before and after my workout, and in the morning when I first wake up.

Supplements to Balance Your pH

ALKAMIND

getoffyouracid.com

My buddy Daryl Gioffre, a self-proclaimed former sugar addict, has perfected nutritional strategies for balancing out your body's pH level. The American diet is 90 percent acidic according to Gioffre, and a lot of this is due to a diet that is too full of sugar, overly caffeinated drinks, and processed foods. This acid can burn holes in your gut, your joints, and your muscles. Gioffre offers several products that can help replenish your body and get you back in balance. I especially love his daily greens and minerals.

Supplements for Skin and Hair

DR. TESS

liveli.com

Dr. Tess Mauricio, a board-certified dermatologist, and her husband, Dr. James Lee, a Yale- and Stanford-trained anesthesiologist, designed the nutritional support system they call Liveli. These supplement formulas are selected to help you sleep peacefully at night, to restore your nutrition each day, and to help focus and clear your mind.

Supplements for a Healthy Gut

JJ VIRGIN

jjvirgin.com

Celebrity nutrition and fitness expert JJ Virgin makes many excellent products. I want to highlight two: the Safety Net supplement and Leaky Gut Support supplement. Safety Net is designed to help your body to limit absorption of starches, support healthy weight loss, suppress your appetite, balance your metabolism, and lower your blood sugar. Altogether, this improves your digestive system. Leaky Gut Support contains glutamine, slippery elm, and many other natural ingredients to help heal your gut. If you are experiencing symptoms like gas and bloating, joint pain, fatigue, headaches, acne, and are having trouble losing weight, give this supplement a try.

Sleep Support

NATURAL VITALITY

naturalvitality.com

This company is committed to "calmness," and in our stressed-out 24/7 society, it's a welcome message. One of their product offerings is called Natural Calm. It's a magnesium and calcium powder concentrate that is sweetened with stevia and comes unflavored and also in a variety of fruity flavors. Natural Vitality also has a transdermal magnesium cream called Calm Cream for tense or stiff muscles.

Respiratory Health

XLEAR

xlear.com

Xlear is a natural saline spray made with xylitol, an ingredient that is great at cleaning and moisturizing your sinuses. Standard saline sprays can be drying and leave your nose more irritated instead of less. With Xlear, you'll alleviate congestion and prevent bacteria and other pollutants in your nasal tissues.

GEAR AND EQUIPMENT

Kitchen Equipment

BLENDTEC

blendtec.com

The Blendtec blender is incredibly powerful, and it handles hot and cold items better than any other blender I've ever tried. Enjoy soups, beverages, sauces, condiments, and smoothies. You won't need to unjam the Blendtec every time you're trying to whip up a few ice cubes or some frozen fruit. The power of this blender makes it able to pulverize even the hardest and most challenging of substances. I highly recommend that you give it a try.

Fitness, Health, and Wellness Gear

VASPER

vasper.com

On the Vasper system you sit on what looks sort of like a recumbent bike/elliptical thing that has both hand and foot pedals. Before you begin, your arms and legs are also put in what looks like blood pressure cuffs that use a combination of compression and liquid cooling as you work out. Athletes rave about how they can build better hormone balance and lean tissue, and recover from a workout faster with Vasper. It takes just twenty-one minutes.

KETTLEBELL KINGS

kettlebellkings.com

These are my favorite kettlebells because they come with a softer, smoother finish and are made with more care than others I've used. Plus, you can order them and get free shipping. When I train clients, I always use these kettlebells for toning up. When you are ready to take your Cruise Control Workout to the next level, consider buying a couple of these.

YOYO MATS

yoyomats.com

You know those little slap bracelets that are a classic kids' party favor? They lie straight and then "slap" and curl around your wrist. That's sort of how YoYo Mats were designed. These innovative mats roll out straight and then, with a flip at the end of class, they self-roll back up.

SPRI

spri.com

Spri sells just about everything that has to do with fitness and wellness. Stability balls, mats, medicine balls, exercise bands, dumbbells, weighted bars, jump ropes, plyoboxes, and more. If you are looking for fitness equipment, look here.

MYOBUDDY

myobuddy.com

"Oh my goodness!" That seems to be the most common response when people get to try this new heated self-massager. The MyoBuddy is a percussive massager that places professional-grade deep tissue warming to increase blood circulation, soothe stiff and sore muscles, and offer wellness in seconds.

GRAVITY BLANKETS

gravityblankets.com

These super-soft weighted blankets improve sleep and reduce stress and anxiety by making you feel as if you are being held or hugged. We sleep with our Gravity Blankets every night, and we also love to cuddle with them when we watch TV.

FITNESS, HEALTH, AND WELLNESS CENTERS

EQUINOX

equinox.com

These club memberships come with personal training, yoga, cycling, Barre classes, Pilates, and more. They provide towels and locker rooms and have a juice bar and spa. Many of these establishments have childcare, and they often have cafés and lounges.

24 HOUR FITNESS

24hourfitness.com

This nationwide gym chain is perfect for people who are looking to get results with my Belly Burning plan and get happy and healthy with whatever makes you feel good, whether that's weight lifting, classes, cardio, or laps in the pool. Whether you're a busy mom or grandparent, professional athlete or weekend warrior, you'll find a community of people like you, working at their own pace to reach their goals. The best workout is the one that you'll stick to, and 24 Hour Fitness offers plenty of options, including strength and cardio equipment, fitness classes, personal training, basketball courts, turf zones, swimming pools, saunas, and whirlpools. (Don't make kids an excuse not to take time for your health—many locations have kids' clubs, too.) You'll even receive a free personalized fitness plan created by a certified trainer featuring customized workouts that you can do in club and that are available through the free 24 GO app—along with hundreds more workouts—so you always know what to do and how to do it, whether you're in the gym or on the go.

PULSE CENTERS

pulsecenters.com

At Pulse Centers, you'll find a machine that works to charge up your cells. Called pulsed electromagnetic fields (PEMF) technology, it improves your body's energy production, oxygenation, circulation, hydration, and detoxification and gives your body the ability to absorb nutrients better.

JOOVV

joovv.com

Using next-level light therapy, Joovv helps you reach your health and fitness goals by encouraging weight loss, muscle recovery, and skin health while reducing joint pain, hormone imbalances, and inflammation. Joovv uses red and near-infrared light, which allows oxygen to bind to other elements to help your body produce energy. It's this energy production that enhances cellular performance.

SUNLIGHTEN SAUNAS

sunlighten.com

Sunlighten Saunas provide your own at-home sauna, so you have a place to heal, reflect, and invest in yourself. These saunas promote natural healing by penetrating human tissue, which in turn produces a host of antiaging health benefits. It's one of the "hottest" home therapies available.

NANOVI
eng3corp.com

This device provides a signal that helps damaged cells repair and fights the damage of free radicals. NanoVi at-home products generate a specific electromagnetic wave to help your body naturally repair cell damage and counteract the effects of harmful reactive oxygen species.

CRYO
cryousasolutions.com

CryoUSA is a top supplier of whole-body cryotherapy units and other recovery products. Cryotherapy uses extreme cooling on the body that helps to reduce systemwide pain and inflammation. New research is also showing the benefits of using cryotherapy to reduce stress and anxiety.

SAMINA
saminasleep.com

Healthy sleep is essential for your body and your trillions of cells to rest, repair, and replenish. Samina sleep products range from pillows, to bedding, to mattresses. Samina uses the highest-quality all-natural materials to promote healthy sleep.

SYNERGY SCIENCE
synergyscience.com

Synergy Science provides machines that deliver purified, pH-balanced, and hydrogen-enriched water, which has been shown to reduce cell-damaging free radicals that can cause disease and cancers.

TRUEDARK
truedark.com

These glasses by TrueDark are sold in a pack of two pairs, one for the day and another for nighttime. The lenses in these glasses help to reset your natural circadian rhythm by reducing your exposure to the artificial or "junk" light that is now part of our 24/7 lifestyles. This junk light may contribute to eye strain, headaches, memory loss, insomnia, stress, anxiety, and more.

CVAC

cvacsysystems.com

A Cyclic Variations in Adaptive Conditioning (CVAC) pod is an elliptical self-enclosed machine that enhances high performance by simulating a high-altitude environment. How? It pulls air out of the pod to create the sort of thinner air that you'd get at higher altitudes, to improve lung capacity and reduce pain, according to some studies.

APPS

These are available on your iPhone, iPad, or iPod touch app store.

Zero: A simple fasting tracker, Zero can be used for intermittent, circadian rhythm, and custom fasting. You can choose the window that suits you, and Zero will track your ongoing progress on your iPhone or Apple Watch. You can export data to a spreadsheet as well.

Breathe: The Breathe app works on your Apple Watch to guide you through a series of deep breaths and reminds you to take time to breathe every day. Customizable to your individual preferences.

Brooke Burke Body: Join Brooke Burke, celebrity health and wellness guru, on her bite-size workouts for all fitness levels. You can choose to work on getting flat toned abs, lean and firm legs, or a whole-body makeover. Available on iPhone, iPad, and iPod touch.

My Fitness by Jillian Michaels: Daily seven-minute workouts with fitness star Jillian Michaels. Here you'll find videos with clear instructions and lots of encouragement. Also available are calorie counters, weight-loss programs, and an advanced meal planner system.

Sweat: Kayla Itsines Fitness: Join the world's biggest female fitness community and fast-track your journey to a better body. This app includes twenty-eight-minute workouts, customizable meal plans, and other fitness challenges. There are also programs for yoga, weights, and post-pregnancy workouts.

Headspace: This meditation app shows you how to reframe stress with guided meditations and mindfulness techniques that bring calm, wellness, and balance to your life in just a few minutes a day. Also included are meditations that help you to relax and sleep better at night.

MyFitnessPal: An app that will help you to keep track of your eating, allow you to look up nutrition information on more than six million foods, quickly scan barcodes for nutrition information, and help you with your goals to lose weight, tone up, get healthy, or create a new habit.

PODCASTS

The Cruise Control Podcast: Put yourself in the driver's seat of your health and wellness with Hollywood trainer and #1 *New York Times* bestselling author Jorge Cruise. Listen in as Jorge guides you on your journey to total health. In each episode, you'll find a mix of weekly inspiration and entertainment, including interviews with celebrities, doctors, thought leaders, trainers, and influencers.

The Skinny Confidential Him & Her Podcast: Lauryn Evarts Bosstick and Michael Bosstick, entrepreneurs and brand builders, bring you a mix of celebrity interviews, experts, and thought leaders. Listener Q&As are addressed each week regarding health, wellness, business, branding, marketing, and relationships.

Aubrey Marcus: The founder of Onnit and author of *Own the Day,* modern philosopher Aubrey Marcus discusses the important questions: How do we find our purpose, wake up to who we truly are, not take ourselves so seriously, and live life a little better?

Mindbodygreen Podcast: Hear motivational interviews with experts who are shaping a whole new wellness world by including the wisdom of healing practices from all over the world. These cutting-edge thinkers are interviewed by Jason Wachob, founder and CEO of mindbodygreen, in a casual, relaxed setting. You'll hear personal journeys, struggles, and how these experts have overcome obstacles.

The Jillian Michaels Show: This is a new inspirational and informative show to help you find health and happiness in all areas of your life. A new episode is out every Monday. Join Jillian and her crew as they have conversations with her favorite experts and friends about fitness, well-being, and much more.

America's Doctor: The Dr. Oz Podcast: Listen as Dr. Mehmet Oz interviews world leaders, authors, and other health and wellness experts on their strategies and techniques for exploring health secrets, wellness tips, and design for living a better life.

The Intermittent Fasting Podcast: Authors Melanie Avalon (*The What When Wine Diet: Paleo and Intermittent Fasting for Health and Weight Loss*) and Gin Stephens (*Delay, Don't Deny: Living an Intermittent Fasting Lifestyle*) bring their personal experiences with intermittent fasting, discuss the one-meal-a-day lifestyle, and tell how intermittent fasting has helped them to lose weight and be healthier overall.

Primal Blueprint Podcast: On how to be healthy, strong, fit, and happy, with the least amount of pain, suffering, and sacrifice possible. Featuring *Primal Blueprint* author Mark Sisson (marksdailyapple.com) and other guests from the ancestral health community.

SHARING SUCCESS ON CRUISE CONTROL

Please send me your before-and-after photos, your Cruise Control–related victories, and personal triumphs on your journey toward health and wellness. Your health success is my passion—honestly! I want to hear about it, and there are various ways you can share your Cruise Control story with me, including facebook.com/jorgecruise; on Instagram at @jorgecruise, #CruiseControlDiet, and #JorgeCruise. Want to stay private? No problem. I'll secure your expressed permission before using any part of your story, and if you want to keep it between just the two of us, that's okay, too.

FINDING A CRUISE CONTROL–FRIENDLY MEDICAL PRACTITIONER

I highly recommend finding a health practitioner who takes all of the world's many healing philosophies into account. By honoring who you are as an individual with unique biology and life circumstances, that's what integrative and functional medicine do. Integrative medicine honors all healing practices as long as they have scientific evidence backing their credibility. Functional medicine addresses the underlying causes of disease by spending time with patients to collect a full history and to understand the genetic, environmental, and lifestyle factors that can influence physical, mental, and emotional health.

Here are three websites that will help you find a health practitioner that's right for you in your location:

Institute for Functional Medicine: ifm.org

The American Board of Integrative Holistic Medicine: abihm.org/search-doctors

Integrative Medicine for Mental Health: integrativemedicineformentalhealth.com/registry.php

And a final shout-out to two fantastic health experts: These are docs who have helped me personally. A phenomenal expert in dental health and another, an innovator in skin health. Both have introduced me to new science in both of these areas. If you are lucky enough to live close to either, I highly recommend that you seek their healing wisdom:

Dental Health
DR. GABE ROSENTHAL
gaberosenthaldds.com

Is this a shameless plug for my dentist? It is, but for a good reason. Let's face it, your dentist is second only to your hairstylist (once you find a good one, you stay put). Dr. Gabe grew up in Southern California, and he's been our go-to dental health expert for my entire family. I know that not everyone lives in Southern California (where Dr. Gabe is located), but he has a great blog that answers just about any question you might have regarding crowns, whitening, cosmetic dentistry, root canals, dental implants, and more. Dr. Gabe comes from a family of dentists, and he started by volunteering his time while in college, assisting other dentists and helping people who were living in underserved communities.

Dr. Gabe's father, Leslie Rosenthal, has been a dentist in Encino for four decades. Together, they have collaborated on many complex cosmetic and restorative dental cases. Dr. Gabe's sister, Erica, is a dental hygienist. The family works side by side to provide comprehensive dental care for their patients. After Dr. Gabe graduated from the USC School of Dentistry (with honors, of course), he worked for the USC Sports Dental Program as a student dentist. During this time, Dr. Gabe treated many student athletes who have gone on to play for the NBA and NFL.

Dr. Gabe serves as the Cosmetic, Invisalign, and CAD/CAM (same-day-crowns) expert for the Katz Dental Group in the Los Angeles/ Beverly Hills office. If you're long overdue for a cleaning, or you are interested in Invisalign, the clear alternative to braces, Dr. Gabe can answer your questions.

Skin Health

DR. DEEPAK DUGAR

scarlessnose.com

Dr. Dugar has dedicated his entire career to helping patients turn back the clock on aging. He is known for his artistry with subtle nose jobs, skin treatments, and other procedures. Dr. Dugar's patients travel from around the world seeking his help. At his clinic, he offers both nonsurgical and surgical cosmetic procedures that help you finesse your face and body to be beautiful. He also supports the use of natural supplements to improve your skin health to help you look years younger.

Dr. Dugar's research in the medical field has been published in internationally acclaimed peer-reviewed journals, and he continues to lecture and teach at national medical conferences around the country. Dr. Dugar's philosophy on nonsurgical procedures is the same as considering plastic surgery. You must always analyze the risk vs. the benefit ratio. Dr. Dugar is a trusted medical expert used by ABC News, E! News, and *HuffPost,* where he routinely serves as a medical adviser on the latest and greatest cosmetic procedures used by Hollywood celebrities.

If you've been thinking about fixing loose skin, dark circles around your eyes, or even hair renewal and regrowth procedures, you'll find lots of helpful information and services available at Dr. Dugar's site.

ACKNOWLEDGMENTS

I am so grateful to all the wonderful, talented people at Ballantine Books, with special thanks to the brilliant Marnie Cochran, my marvelous editor, as well as the rest of the Ballantine team: Kara Welsh, Kim Hovey, Jennifer Hershey, Leigh Marchant, Cindy Murray, Debbie Aroff, Stacy Horowitz, Joe Perez, and Hanna Gibeau.

Thank you to my agent, Byrd Leavell, my publicist, British Reece, and my manager, David Brady, and thank you so much to my number one mentor and supporter, Raymond Garcia.

Of course, the biggest thanks goes to my sons, Parker Cruise and Owen Cruise, for always having your dad's back. I love you boys more than you'll ever know and can't wait for the adventures ahead.

Special thanks to you Sam J. Ayers; thank you for all your support and love during the past five years. When I needed you, you were there for me and I will always remember that. An extra special thank you for helping collaborate with me on the delicious meals in this book. Please know I am here for you, too.

A book may credit only one author on the cover, but anyone who has ever worked on a manuscript knows that it takes a village. I am blessed to have an amazingly gifted, creative, and brilliant team of researchers, writers, editors, fact-checkers, and assistants. Thank you to Alex Watson, my right-hand man and ninja *extraordinaire* (you make my life easier in so many ways), and also to Marianne M. Kotcher (my masterful word-smith), Stephen Steigler, and Deborah Feingold.

I also couldn't have done this book without the cutting-edge experts who took the time to let me pick their brains. Thank you, Dr. Andrew Weil, Mark Sisson, Dr. Jason Fung, Brooke Burke, Aubrey Marcus, Naomi Whittel, Dr. Cate Shanahan, Dr. Daryl Gioffre, and Dr. Satchin Panda.

Another essential component of shaping this book were the thousands of test panelists who took on Cruise Control, saw life-changing results, and gave feedback to help fine-tune and develop the Cruise Control lifestyle in these pages.

There are so many other people who offered their support, feedback, and time. Thank you for contributing your advice, knowledge, and support. While this list could go on and on, I wish to thank a few of my friends here:

Steve Harvey	Jillian Michaels	Aaron Rapoport
Terence Noonan	Khloe Kardashian	Gabrielle Reece
Jeff Williams	Jameel Spencer	Cameron Mathison
Jay Blahnik	Keith Frankel	Brianna Campbell
Richard Galanti	Sandie Renfrow	Laird Hamilton
Pennie Clark	Noah Gelbart	Jessica Simpson
Ianniciello	JJ Virgin	Edward Ash-Milby
Mary Ellen Keating	Kayla Itsines	Oprah Winfrey
Leslie Marcus	Jeanette Jenkins	Sandy Torrey
John Redmann	Marco Borges	Jennifer Lopez
Lisa Gregorisch-	Rachael Ray	Tim Talevich
Dempsey	Dr. Deepak Dugar	Tyra Banks
Carol Brooks	Dr. Howard Leibowitz	Heather Spangler
James Avenell	Dr. Gabe Rosenthal	Alex Duda
Natalie Bubnis	Katie Couric	Suzanne Somers
Scott Eason	Bobbi Brown	Emeril Lagasse
Lisa Wheeler	Lashaun Dale	Lucy Lui
Dr. Mehmet Oz	David Harris	Mario Lopez
Dr. David Katz	Luann de Lesseps	Roni Selig
Jacqui Stafford	Joan and Rick Ayers	Dorinda Medley
Al Roker	Sterling Chase	Candi Carter
Anthony Robbins	Mazeratie Sweet	Jeff Williams
Bruce Barlean	Amy Mullen	Julz Arney
Cathy Chermol	Loan Dang	Craig Bolton
Janet Annino	Mel Mauer	Barrie Galanti
Hilary Estey	Jen Brookman	Stephen Perrine
McLoughlin	Beth Sobol	Bob Love
Marta Fox	Patricia Ciano	Jane Francisco
Stephen Steigler	Dr. Tess Mauricio	Steve Morris
Brooke Burke	Khalil Rafati	Julissa Soriano

Toby Reiter
Stuart K. Robinson
Brandon Aristotle
    Lucas
Stewart Volland
Dr. Jason Fung
Mark Sisson

And special thanks to:

Ross Taylor
Kara Taylor
Chris Roussos
Tom Lapcevic
Andress Blackwell
Alfonso Tejada
Scott Nelson
Elizabeth Nelson
Justin Strahan

Melissa Strahan
Wes Pfiffner
Brian Hemmert
Jeffrey Frese
Andy Barbera
Lisa Jubilee
Aspen Lewis
Mason Arnold
Amy Lacey
Ellen Yin
Jimi Sturgeon-Smith
Kevin Joseph
Holly Richardson
Mike McAdams
Kris Saim-Gentry
Jason Lincoln Jeffers
Jenny Chen
Pete Maldonado
Louis Armstrong

Kris Altiere
Greg Johnson
Emilio Palafox
Rowena Gates
Hans Eng
Evan Sims
Claus Pummer
Denise Pummer
Nathan Jones
Jay Perkins
Amir Amirsadeghi
Mike Apostal
Sebastian Wasowski
Peter Wasowski
Michael Mulcahy
Heath Squier
Cheney Squier

SELECTED BIBLIOGRAPHY

CHAPTER 1: TIMING IS EVERYTHING

Asif, Mohammad. "The Prevention and Control of Type-2 Diabetes by Changing Lifestyle and Dietary Pattern." *Journal of Education and Health Promotion* 3, no. 1 (2014): 1. https://doi.org/10.4103/2277-9531.127541.

Bluher, M. "Extended Longevity in Mice Lacking the Insulin Receptor in Adipose Tissue." *Science* 299, no. 5606 (01, 2003): 572–74. https://doi.org/10.1126/science.1078223.

Bueno, Nassib Bezerra, et al. "Very-low-carbohydrate Ketogenic Diet v. Low-Fat Diet for Long-Term Weight Loss: A Meta-analysis of Randomised Controlled Trials." *British Journal of Nutrition* 110, no. 07 (05, 2013): 1178–87. https://doi.org/10.1017/s0007114513000548.

Claesson, Anna-Lena, et al. "Two Weeks of Overfeeding with Candy, but Not Peanuts, Increases Insulin Levels and Body Weight." *Scandinavian Journal of Clinical and Laboratory Investigation* 69, no. 5 (01, 2009): 598–605. https://doi.org/10.1080/00365510902912754.

"Comparison of Diets for Weight Loss and Heart Disease Risk Reduction." *JAMA* 293, no. 13 (04, 2005): 1589. https://doi.org/10.1001/jama.293.13.1590-a.

Elliott, Sharon S., et al. "Fructose, Weight Gain, and the Insulin Resistance Syndrome." *The American Journal of Clinical Nutrition* 76, no. 5 (11, 2002): 911–22. https://doi.org/10.1093/ajcn/76.5.911.

Evans, M., et al. "A Review of Modern Insulin Analogue Pharmacokinetic and Pharmacodynamic Profiles in Type 2 Diabetes: Improvements and Limitations." *Diabetes, Obesity and Metabolism* 13, no. 8 (06, 2011): 677–84. https://doi.org/10.1111/j.1463-1326.2011.01395.x.

Franz, Marion, et al. "Evidence-Based Diabetes Nutrition Therapy Recommendations Are Effective: The Key Is Individualization." *Diabetes, Metabolic Syn-

drome and Obesity: Targets and Therapy 2014 (02, 2014): 65. https://doi.org/10.2147/dmso.s45140.

Fung, Jason, and Jimmy Moore. *The Complete Guide to Fasting: Heal Your Body through Intermittent, Alternate-Day, and Extended Fasting.* Victory Belt Publishing, 2016.

Gardner, Christopher D., et al. "Effect of Low-Fat vs Low-Carbohydrate Diet on 12-Month Weight Loss in Overweight Adults and the Association with Genotype Pattern or Insulin Secretion." *JAMA* 319, no. 7 (02, 2018): 667. https://doi.org/10.1001/jama.2018.0245.

Heilbronn, Leonie K., and Eric Ravussin. "Calorie Restriction and Aging: Review of the Literature and Implications for Studies in Humans." *The American Journal of Clinical Nutrition* 78, no. 3 (09, 2003): 361–69. https://doi.org/10.1093/ajcn/78.3.361.

Henry, R. R., et al. "Intensive Conventional Insulin Therapy for Type II Diabetes: Metabolic Effects during a 6-mo Outpatient Trial." *Diabetes Care* 16, no. 1 (01, 1993): 21–31. https://doi.org/10.2337/diacare.16.1.21.

Holman, Rury R., et al. "Addition of Biphasic, Prandial, or Basal Insulin to Oral Therapy in Type 2 Diabetes." *New England Journal of Medicine* 357, no. 17 (10, 2007): 1716–30. https://doi.org/10.1056/nejmoa075392.

Ibero-Baraibar, Idoia, et al. "Different Postprandial Acute Response in Healthy Subjects to Three Strawberry Jams Varying in Carbohydrate and Antioxidant Content: A Randomized, Crossover Trial." *European Journal of Nutrition* 53, no. 1 (04, 2013): 201–10. https://doi.org/10.1007/s00394-013-0517-7.

"Insulin Basics." American Diabetes Association. http://www.diabetes.org/living-with-diabetes/treatment-and-care/medication/insulin/insulin-basics.html?referrer=https://www.google.com/.

"Insulin Resistance & Prediabetes." National Institute of Diabetes and Digestive and Kidney Diseases. May 1, 2018. https://www.niddk.nih.gov/health-information/diabetes/overview/what-is-diabetes/prediabetes-insulin-resistance.

Kalra, Sanjay, and Jeffrey L. Roitman. "Comparison of the Atkins, Zone, Ornish, and Learn Diets for Change in Weight and Related Risk Factors among Overweight Premenopausal Women." *Journal of Cardiopulmonary Rehabilitation and Prevention* 27, no. 4 (07, 2007): 254–55. https://doi.org/10.1097/01.hcr.0000281777.02845.22.

Keller, Ulrich. "Dietary Proteins in Obesity and in Diabetes." *International Journal for Vitamin and Nutrition Research* 81, no. 23 (03, 2011): 125–33. https://doi.org/10.1024/0300-9831/a000059.

Kong, Ling Chun, et al. "Insulin Resistance and Inflammation Predict Kinetic Body Weight Changes in Response to Dietary Weight Loss and Maintenance in Overweight and Obese Subjects by Using a Bayesian Network Approach." *The American Journal of Clinical Nutrition* 98, no. 6 (10, 2013): 1385–94. https://doi.org/10.3945/ajcn.113.058099.

Lebovitz, H. "Insulin Resistance: Definition and Consequences." *Experimental and Clinical Endocrinology & Diabetes* 109, no. Suppl 2 (11, 2001): S135–S148. https://doi.org/10.1055/s-2001-18576.

Lin, Wei-Ting, et al. "Fructose-Rich Beverage Intake and Central Adiposity, Uric Acid, and Pediatric Insulin Resistance." *The Journal of Pediatrics* 171 (04, 2016): 90–96. https://doi.org/10.1016/j.jpeds.2015.12.061.

Panda, Satchin. *The Circadian Code: Lose Weight, Supercharge Your Energy, and Transform Your Health from Morning to Midnight.* Rodale, 2018.

Raatz, Susan K., et al. "Consumption of Honey, Sucrose, and High-Fructose Corn Syrup Produces Similar Metabolic Effects in Glucose-Tolerant and -Intolerant Individuals." *The Journal of Nutrition* 145, no. 10 (09, 2015): 2265–72. https://doi.org/10.3945/jn.115.218016.

Raben, Anne, et al. "Increased Postprandial Glycaemia, Insulinemia, and Lipidemia after 10 Weeks' Sucrose-Rich Diet Compared to an Artificially Sweetened Diet: A Randomised Controlled Trial." *Food & Nutrition Research* 55, no. 1 (01, 2011): 5961. https://doi.org/10.3402/fnr.v55i0.5961.

Rizkalla, Salwa W. "Health Implications of Fructose Consumption: A Review of Recent Data." *Nutrition & Metabolism* 7, no. 1 (2010): 82. https://doi.org/10.1186/1743-7075-7-82.

Rolls, B. J. "What Is the Role of Portion Control in Weight Management?" *International Journal of Obesity* 38, no. S1 (07, 2014): S1–S8. https://doi.org/10.1038/ijo.2014.82.

Sacks, Frank M., et al. "Comparison of Weight-Loss Diets with Different Compositions of Fat, Protein, and Carbohydrates." *Obstetrical & Gynecological Survey* 64, no. 7 (07, 2009): 460–62. https://doi.org/10.1097/01.ogx.0000351673.32059.13.

Stanhope, Kimber L., et al. "Consuming Fructose-Sweetened, Not Glucose-Sweetened, Beverages Increases Visceral Adiposity and Lipids and Decreases Insulin Sensitivity in Overweight/Obese Humans." *Journal of Clinical Investigation* 119, no. 5 (05, 2009): 1322–34. https://doi.org/10.1172/jci37385.

Steyn, N. P., et al. "Diet, Nutrition and the Prevention of Type 2 Diabetes." *Public Health Nutrition* 7, no. 1a (02, 2004): 147–165. https://doi.org/10.1079/phn2003586.

Trepanowski, John F., et al. "Impact of Caloric and Dietary Restriction Regimens on Markers of Health and Longevity in Humans and Animals: A Summary of Available Findings." *Nutrition Journal* 10, no. 1 (10, 2011): 107. https://doi.org/10.1186/1475-2891-10-107.

Varady, K. A. "Intermittent versus Daily Calorie Restriction: Which Diet Regimen Is More Effective for Weight Loss?" *Obesity Reviews* 12, no. 7 (03, 2011): e593–601. https://doi.org/10.1111/j.1467-789x.2011.00873.x.

CHAPTER 2: TURNING ON CRUISE CONTROL AND STARTING TO BURN

Acheson, K. J., et al. "Caffeine and Coffee: Their Influence on Metabolic Rate and Substrate Utilization in Normal Weight and Obese Individuals." *The American Journal of Clinical Nutrition* 33, no. 5 (05, 1980): 989–97. https://doi.org/10.1093/ajcn/33.5.989.

Cunnane, Stephen C., et al. "Can Ketones Compensate for Deteriorating Brain Glucose Uptake during Aging? Implications for the Risk and Treatment of Alzheimer's Disease." *Annals of the New York Academy of Sciences* 1367, no. 1 (01, 2016): 12–20. https://doi.org/10.1111/nyas.12999.

Doherty, M., and P. M. Smith. "Effects of Caffeine Ingestion on Rating of Perceived Exertion during and after Exercise: A Meta-analysis." *Scandinavian Journal of Medicine and Science in Sports* 15, no. 2 (04, 2005): 69–78. https://doi.org/10.1111/j.1600-0838.2005.00445.x.

Gabel, Kelsey, et al. "Safety of 8-h Time Restricted Feeding in Adults with Obesity." *Applied Physiology, Nutrition, and Metabolism* (09, 2018). https://doi.org/10.1139/apnm-2018-0389.

Hatori, Megumi, et al. "Time-Restricted Feeding without Reducing Caloric Intake Prevents Metabolic Diseases in Mice Fed a High-Fat Diet." *Cell Metabolism* 15, no. 6 (06, 2012): 848–60. https://doi.org/10.1016/j.cmet.2012.04.019.

Henning, Susanne M., et al. "Decaffeinated Green and Black Tea Polyphenols Decrease Weight Gain and Alter Microbiome Populations and Function in Diet-Induced Obese Mice." *European Journal of Nutrition* 57, no. 8 (12, 2018): 2759–69. https://doi.org/10.1007/s00394-017-1542-8.

Mattson, Mark P., et al. "Impact of Intermittent Fasting on Health and Disease Processes." *Ageing Research Reviews* 39 (10, 2017): 46–58. https://doi.org/10.1016/j.arr.2016.10.005.

Melkani, Girish C., and Satchidananda Panda. "Time-Restricted Feeding for Prevention and Treatment of Cardiometabolic Disorders." *The Journal of Physiology* 595, no. 12 (04, 2017): 3691–700. https://doi.org/10.1113/jp273094.

Panda, Satchin. *The Circadian Code: Lose Weight, Supercharge Your Energy, and Transform Your Health from Morning to Midnight.* Rodale, 2018.

Ruxton, C. H. S. "The Impact of Caffeine on Mood, Cognitive Function, Performance and Hydration: A Review of Benefits and Risks." *Nutrition Bulletin* 33, no. 1 (03, 2008): 15–25. https://doi.org/10.1111/j.1467-3010.2007.00665.x.

"10 Reasons to Drink Green Tea—Dr. Weil's Healthy Kitchen." DrWeil.com. October 9, 2017. https://www.drweil.com/diet-nutrition/nutrition/10-reasons-to-drink-green-tea/.

Vandenberghe, Camille, et al. "Caffeine Intake Increases Plasma Ketones: An Acute Metabolic Study in Humans." *Canadian Journal of Physiology and Pharmacology* 95, no. 4 (04, 2017): 455–58. https://doi.org/10.1139/cjpp-2016-0338.

Vogel, Leanne. *The Keto Diet: The Complete Guide to a High-Fat Diet, with More than 125 Delectable Recipes and 5 Meal Plans to Shed Weight, Heal Your Body & Regain Confidence.* Victory Belt Publishing, 2017.

CHAPTER 3: GET A BOOST: EATING MATTERS, TOO

Atkins, Robert C. *Dr. Atkins' Nutrition Breakthrough: How to Treat Your Medical Condition without Drugs.* Bantam Books, 1988.

Banting, William. *Letter on Corpulence, Addressed to the Public: With a Review of the Work from Blackwood's . . . Magazine, and an Article on Corpulency Leanness Fr.* Forgotten Books, 2017.

Banting, William. *Letter on Corpulence, Addressed to the Public.* Harrison, 1885.

Betts, James A., et al. "The Causal Role of Breakfast in Energy Balance and Health: A Randomized Controlled Trial in Lean Adults." *The American Journal of Clinical Nutrition* 100, no. 2 (06, 2014): 539–47. https://doi.org/10.3945/ajcn.114.083402.

Blondeau, Nicolas, et al. "Alpha-Linolenic Acid: An Omega-3 Fatty Acid with Neuroprotective Properties—Ready for Use in the Stroke Clinic?" *BioMed Research International* 2015 (2015): 1–8. https://doi.org/10.1155/2015/519830.

Carreiro, Alicia L., et al. "The Macronutrients, Appetite, and Energy Intake." *Annual Review of Nutrition* 36, no. 1 (07, 2016): 73–103. https://doi.org/10.1146/annurev-nutr-121415-112624.

Carroll, Abigail. *Three Squares: The Invention of the American Meal*. Basic Books, a Member of the Perseus Books Group, 2013.

Dhaka, Vandana, et al. "Trans Fats—Sources, Health Risks and Alternative Approach—A Review." *Journal of Food Science and Technology* 48, no. 5 (01, 2011): 534–41. https://doi.org/10.1007/s13197-010-0225-8.

Flegal, Katherine M., et al. "Prevalence of Obesity and Trends in the Distribution of Body Mass Index Among US Adults, 1999–2010." *JAMA* 307, no. 5 (02, 2012): 491. https://doi.org/10.1001/jama.2012.39.

Ibero-Baraibar, Idoia, et al. "Different Postprandial Acute Response in Healthy Subjects to Three Strawberry Jams Varying in Carbohydrate and Antioxidant Content: A Randomized, Crossover Trial." *European Journal of Nutrition* 53, no. 1 (04, 2013): 201–10. https://doi.org/10.1007/s00394-013-0517-7.

"Is Breakfast the Most Important Meal?" PBS. https://www.pbs.org/video/is-breakfast-the-most-important-meal-xas6ug/.

Katan, M. B. "Trans-Fatty Acids and Their Effects on Lipoproteins in Humans." *Annual Review of Nutrition* 15, no. 1 (01, 1995): 473–93. https://doi.org/10.1146/annurev.nutr.15.1.473.

Kim, Il-Young, et al. "Quantity of Dietary Protein Intake, but Not Pattern of Intake, Affects Net Protein Balance Primarily through Differences in Protein Synthesis in Older Adults." *American Journal of Physiology-Endocrinology and Metabolism* 308, no. 1 (01, 2015): E21–E28. https://doi.org/10.1152/ajpendo.00382.2014.

Lopez-Huertas, Eduardo. "Health Effects of Oleic Acid and Long Chain Omega-3 Fatty Acids (EPA and DHA) Enriched Milks. A Review of Intervention Studies." *Pharmacological Research* 61, no. 3 (03, 2010): 200–207. https://doi.org/10.1016/j.phrs.2009.10.007.

Mackarness, Richard. *Eat Fat and Grow Slim*. www.bnpublishing.com, 2017.

McCarty, Mark F., and James J. Dinicolantonio. "Lauric Acid-Rich Medium-Chain Triglycerides Can Substitute for Other Oils in Cooking Applications and May Have Limited Pathogenicity." *Open Heart* 3, no. 2 (07, 2016): e000467. https://doi.org/10.1136/openhrt-2016-000467.

Mensink, Ronald P. "Effects of Stearic Acid on Plasma Lipid and Lipoproteins in Humans." *Lipids* 40, no. 12 (12, 2005): 1201–05. https://doi.org/10.1007/s11745-005-1486-x.

Mozaffarian, Dariush, et al. "Changes in Diet and Lifestyle and Long-Term Weight Gain in Women and Men." *New England Journal of Medicine* 364, no. 25 (06, 2011): 2392–404. https://doi.org/10.1056/nejmoa1014296.

Mozaffarian, Dariush, et al. "Dietary Intake of Trans Fatty Acids and Systemic Inflammation in Women." *The American Journal of Clinical Nutrition* 79, no. 4 (04, 2004): 606–12. https://doi.org/10.1093/ajcn/79.4.606.

"Nutrition." Centers for Disease Control and Prevention. May 12, 2017. https://www.cdc.gov/nutrition/data-statistics/plain-water-the-healthier-choice.html.

Oksman, Olga. "How Lobbyists Made Breakfast 'the Most Important Meal of the Day.'" *The Guardian*, November 28, 2016. https://www.theguardian.com/lifeandstyle/2016/nov/28/breakfast-health-america-kellog-food-lifestyle.

Palo, Carlo, et al. "Dietary-induced Thermogenesis in Obesity. Response to Mixed and Carbohydrate Meals." *Acta Diabetologica Latina* 26, no. 2 (06, 1989): 155–62. https://doi.org/10.1007/bf02581367.

Popkin, Barry M., et al. "Water, Hydration, and Health." *Nutrition Reviews* 68, no. 8 (07, 2010): 439–58. https://doi.org/10.1111/j.1753-4887.2010.00304.x.

Reynolds, Gretchen. "Is Breakfast Overrated?" *The New York Times*, August 21, 2014. https://well.blogs.nytimes.com/2014/08/21/is-breakfast-overrated/?_r=0.

Roberts, Susan B., and Gerard E. Dallal. "Energy Requirements and Aging." *Public Health Nutrition* 8, no. 7a (10, 2005): 1028-36. https://doi.org/10.1079/phn2005794.

Russell, Fraser, and Corinna Bürgin-Maunder. "Distinguishing Health Benefits of Eicosapentaenoic and Docosahexaenoic Acids." *Marine Drugs* 10, no. 12 (11, 2012): 2535–559. https://doi.org/10.3390/md10112535.

Schusdziarra, Volker, et al. "Impact of Breakfast on Daily Energy Intake—an Analysis of Absolute versus Relative Breakfast Calories." *Nutrition Journal* 10, no. 1 (01, 2011). https://doi.org/10.1186/1475-2891-10-5.

Sisson, Mark. *Primal Blueprint: Reprogram Your Genes for Effortless Weight Loss, Vibrant Health*. Primal Nutrition, 2012.

Swaminathan, R., et al. "Thermic Effect of Feeding Carbohydrate, Fat, Protein and Mixed Meal in Lean and Obese Subjects." *The American Journal of Clinical Nutrition* 42, no. 2 (08, 1985): 177–81. https://doi.org/10.1093/ajcn/42.2.177.

Tallima, Hatem, and Rashika El Ridi. "Arachidonic Acid: Physiological Roles and Potential Health Benefits—A Review." *Journal of Advanced Research* 11 (05, 2018): 33–41. https://doi.org/10.1016/j.jare.2017.11.004.

Westerterp, Kr, et al. "Diet Induced Thermogenesis Measured over 24h in a Respiration Chamber: Effect of Diet Composition." *International Journal of Obesity* 23, no. 3 (03, 1999): 287–92. https://doi.org/10.1038/sj.ijo.0800810.

Whigham, Leah D., et al. "Efficacy of Conjugated Linoleic Acid for Reducing Fat Mass: A Meta-analysis in Humans." *The American Journal of Clinical Nutrition* 85, no. 5 (05, 2007): 1203–11. https://doi.org/10.1093/ajcn/85.5.1203.

Whigham, Leah D., et al. "Increased Vegetable and Fruit Consumption during Weight Loss Effort Correlates with Increased Weight and Fat Loss." *Nutrition & Diabetes* 2, no. 10 (10, 2012): e48. https://doi.org/10.1038/nutd.2012.22.

Williamson, David F. "Descriptive Epidemiology of Body Weight and Weight Change in U.S. Adults." *Annals of Internal Medicine* 119, no. 7, Part 2 (10, 1993): 646. https://doi.org/10.7326/0003-4819-119-7_part_2-199310011-00004.

Yanovski, Jack A., et al. "A Prospective Study of Holiday Weight Gain." *New England Journal of Medicine* 342, no. 12 (03, 2000): 861–67. https://doi.org/10.1056/nejm200003233421206.

Zinczenko, David, and Peter Moore. *The 8-Hour Diet: Watch the Pounds Disappear without Watching What You Eat!* St. Martin's Press, 2015.

CHAPTER 4: MINDSET & MOTIVATION

Baran, Ben. "Employee Motivation: Goal-Setting Theory." YouTube, January 18, 2012. www.youtube.com/watch?v=_yj2wsPJEWs.

Bokszczanin, Anna. "Social Support Provided by Adolescents Following a Disaster and Perceived Social Support, Sense of Community at School, and Proactive Coping." *Anxiety, Stress & Coping* 25, no. 5 (2012): 575–92. https://doi.org/10.1080/10615806.2011.622374.

Bouskila-Yam, Osnat, and Avraham N. Kluger. "Strength-Based Performance Appraisal and Goal Setting." *Human Resource Management Review* 21, no. 2 (2011): 137–47. https://doi.org/10.1016/j.hrmr.2010.09.001.

"Break the Bonds of Emotional Eating: MedlinePlus Medical Encyclopedia." *MedlinePlus*, U.S. National Library of Medicine. medlineplus.gov/ency/patient instructions/000808.htm.

CartoonStudio. "One-Step-at-a-Time—Goal Achieving Cartoon Doodle Video." YouTube, January 14, 2013. www.youtube.com/watch?v=8cCiqbSJ9fg.

Cascio, Christopher N., et al. "Self-Affirmation Activates Brain Systems Associated with Self-Related Processing and Reward and Is Reinforced by Future Orientation." *Social Cognitive and Affective Neuroscience* 11, no. 4 (05, 2015): 621–29. https://doi.org/10.1093/scan/nsv136.

"Create Your Own Vision Board." *Springboard Beyond Cancer*, July 14, 2017. survivorship.cancer.gov/springboard/get-support/vision-board.

Grav, Siv, et al. "Association between Social Support and Depression in the General Population: The HUNT Study, a Cross-Sectional Survey." *Journal of Clinical Nursing* 21, no. 1–2 (2011): 111–20. https://doi.org/10.1111/j.1365 -2702.2011.03868.x.

"How to Set Your Fitness Goals." *National Institute on Aging*, U.S. Department of Health and Human Services, July 30, 2018. go4life.nia.nih.gov/how-to-set -your-fitness-goals/.

Hwang, Kevin O., et al. "Social Support in an Internet Weight Loss Community." *International Journal of Medical Informatics* 79, no. 1 (2010): 5–13. https:// doi.org/10.1016/j.ijmedinf.2009.10.003.

Janssen, Lieneke K., et al. "Greater Mindful Eating Practice Is Associated with Better Reversal Learning." *Scientific Reports* 8, no. 1 (09, 2018): 5702. https:// doi.org/10.1038/s41598-018-24001-1.

Karfopoulou, Eleni, et al. "The Role of Social Support in Weight Loss Maintenance: Results from the MedWeight Study." *Journal of Behavioral Medicine* 39, no. 3 (2016): 511–18. https://doi.org/10.1007/s10865-016-9717-y.

Miller, Carla K. "Mindful Eating with Diabetes." *Diabetes Spectrum* 30, no. 2 (2017): 89–94. https://doi.org/10.2337/ds16-0039.

Reblin, Maija, and Bert N. Uchino. "Social and Emotional Support and Its Implication for Health." *Current Opinion in Psychiatry* 21, no. 2 (2008): 201–5. https://doi.org/10.1097/yco.0b013e3282f3ad89.

"Study Focuses on Strategies for Achieving Goals, Resolutions." *Dominican University of California*. www.dominican.edu/dominicannews/study-highlights -strategies-forachieving-goals.

Van Strien, Tatjana. "Causes of Emotional Eating and Matched Treatment of Obesity." *Current Diabetes Reports* 18, no. 6 (2018): 35. https://doi.org/10.1007 /s11892-018-1000-x.

Wang, Xingmin, et al. "Social Support Moderates Stress Effects on Depression." *International Journal of Mental Health Systems* 8, no. 1 (2014): 41. https://doi .org/10.1186/1752-4458-8-41.

CHAPTER 5: YOUR FOUR-WEEK PLAN

Ashwell, Margaret, et al. "Waist-to-Height Ratio Is More Predictive of Years of Life Lost than Body Mass Index." *PLoS ONE* 9, no. 9 (08, 2014): e103483. https://doi.org/10.1371/journal.pone.0103483.

Ball, Kylie, et al. "Is Healthy Behavior Contagious: Associations of Social Norms with Physical Activity and Healthy Eating." *International Journal of Behavioral Nutrition and Physical Activity* 7, no. 1 (2010): 86. https://doi.org/10.1186/1479 -5868-7-86.

Chopik, William J., et al. "Changes in Optimism Are Associated with Changes in Health over Time among Older Adults." *Social Psychological and Personality Science* 6, no. 7 (2015): 814–22. https://doi.org/10.1177/1948550615590199.

Conversano, Ciro, et al. "Optimism and Its Impact on Mental and Physical Well-Being." *Clinical Practice & Epidemiology in Mental Health* 1, no. 1 (01, 2010): 25–29. https://doi.org/10.2174/17450179010060100025.

"Excess Fat around the Waist May Increase Death Risk for Women." National Institutes of Health, U.S. Department of Health and Human Services, September 15, 2015. www.nih.gov/news-events/news-releases/excess-fat-around -waist-may-increase-death-risk-women.

Ferdman, Roberto A. "Why Diets Don't Actually Work, According to a Researcher Who Has Studied Them for Decades." *The Washington Post*, May 4, 2015. www.washingtonpost.com/news/wonk/wp/2015/05/04/why-diets-dont -actually-work-according-to-a-researcher-who-has-studied-them-for-decades /?utm_term=.699545a01f54.

Levy, Becca R., et al. "Longevity Increased by Positive Self-Perceptions of Aging." *Journal of Personality and Social Psychology* 83, no. 2 (2002): 261–70. https://doi.org/10.1037//0022-3514.83.2.261.

Mann, Traci, et al. "Medicare's Search for Effective Obesity Treatments: Diets Are Not the Answer." *American Psychologist* 62, no. 3 (2007): 220–33. https://doi.org/10.1037/0003-066x.62.3.220.

Mann, Traci. *Secrets from the Eating Lab: The Science of Weight Loss, the Myth of Willpower, and Why You Should Never Diet Again.* Harper Wave, an imprint of HarperCollins Publishers, 2017.

Mineo, Liz. "Over Nearly 80 Years, Harvard Study Has Been Showing How to Live a Healthy and Happy Life." *Harvard Gazette,* July 24, 2018. news.harvard .edu/gazette/story/2017/04/over-nearly-80-years-harvard-study-has-been -showing-how-to-live-a-healthy-and-happy-life/.

Ozbay, Fatih, et al. "Social Support and Resilience to Stress across the Life Span: A Neurobiologic Framework." *Current Psychiatry Reports* 10, no. 4 (2008): 304– 10. https://doi.org/10.1007/s11920-008-0049-7.

Pillow, David R., et al. "The Need to Belong and Its Association with Fully Satisfying Relationships: A Tale of Two Measures." *Personality and Individual Differences* 74 (2015): 259–64. https://doi.org/10.1016/j.paid.2014.10.031.

Stebleton, Michael J., et al. "First-Generation Students' Sense of Belonging, Mental Health, and Use of Counseling Services at Public Research Universities." *Journal of College Counseling* 17, no. 1 (2014): 6–20. https://doi.org /10.1002/j.2161-1882.2014.00044.x.

Walton, G. M., and G. L. Cohen. "A Brief Social-Belonging Intervention Improves Academic and Health Outcomes of Minority Students." *Science* 331, no. 6023 (2011): 1447–51. https://doi.org/10.1126/science.1198364.

CHAPTER 7: THE EXERCISE EFFECT

Boutcher, Stephen H. "High-Intensity Intermittent Exercise and Fat Loss." *Journal of Obesity* 2011 (2011): 1–10. https://doi.org/10.1155/2011/868305.

Brinke, Lisanne F. Ten, et al. "Aerobic Exercise Increases Hippocampal Volume in Older Women with Probable Mild Cognitive Impairment: A 6-Month Randomised Controlled Trial." *British Journal of Sports Medicine* 49, no. 4 (07, 2014): 248–54. https://doi.org/10.1136/bjsports-2013-093184.

Coelho, Marisa, et al. "State of the Art Paper Biochemistry of Adipose Tissue: An Endocrine Organ." *Archives of Medical Science* 2 (2013): 191–200. https://doi.org/10.5114/aoms.2013.33181.

Fuss, Johannes, et al. "A Runner's High Depends on Cannabinoid Receptors in Mice." *Proceedings of the National Academy of Sciences* 112, no. 42 (05, 2015): 13105–08. https://doi.org/10.1073/pnas.1514996112.

Harvard Health Publishing. "Abdominal Fat and What to Do about It: Visceral Fat More of a Health Concern than Subcutaneous Fat." *Harvard Health.* Published Sept. 2005, updated Oct. 9, 2015.

Phillips, Bill. *Body for Life: 12 Weeks to Mental and Physical Strength.* Harper-Collins, 2003.

Rimer, Jane, et al. "Exercise for Depression." *Cochrane Database of Systematic Reviews*, November 2012. https://doi.org/10.1002/14651858.cd004366.pub5.

Stonerock, Gregory L., et al. "Exercise as Treatment for Anxiety: Systematic Review and Analysis." *Annals of Behavioral Medicine* 49, no. 4 (2015): 542–56. https://doi.org/10.1007/s12160-014-9685-9.

Ströhle, Andreas, et al. "The Acute Antipanic Activity of Aerobic Exercise." *American Journal of Psychiatry* 162, no. 12 (2005): 2376–78. https://doi.org/10.1176/appi.ajp.162.12.2376.

Ströhle, Andreas, et al. "Anxiety Modulation by the Heart? Aerobic Exercise and Atrial Natriuretic Peptide." *Psychoneuroendocrinology* 31, no. 9 (2006): 1127–30. https://doi.org/10.1016/j.psyneuen.2006.08.003.

Zhang, Haifeng, et al. "Comparable Effects of High-Intensity Interval Training and Prolonged Continuous Exercise Training on Abdominal Visceral Fat Reduction in Obese Young Women." *Journal of Diabetes Research* 2017 (2017): 1–9. https://doi.org/10.1155/2017/5071740.

CHAPTER 8: YOUR CRUISE CONTROL WORKOUT

Beavers, Kristen M., et al. "Effect of Exercise Type During Intentional Weight Loss on Body Composition in Older Adults with Obesity." *Obesity* 25, no. 11 (2017): 1823–29. https://doi.org/10.1002/oby.21977.

Beever, Richard. "Do Far-Infrared Saunas Have Cardiovascular Benefits in People with Type 2 Diabetes?" *Canadian Journal of Diabetes* 34, no. 2 (2010): 113–18. https://doi.org/10.1016/s1499-2671(10)42007-9.

Dean, Ward. "Effect of Sweating." *JAMA: The Journal of the American Medical Association* 246, no. 6 (07, 1981): 623. https://doi.org/10.1001/jama.1981 .03320060027013.

Hamblin, Michael R. "Shining Light on the Head: Photobiomodulation for Brain Disorders." *BBA Clinical* 6 (2016): 113–24. https://doi.org/10.1016/j .bbacli.2016.09.002.

Huovinen, Ville, et al. "Bone Mineral Density Is Increased after a 16-Week Resistance Training Intervention in Elderly Women with Decreased Muscle Strength." *European Journal of Endocrinology* 175, no. 6 (2016): 571–82. https:// doi.org/10.1530/eje-16-0521.

Imamura, Masakazu, et al. "Repeated Thermal Therapy Improves Impaired Vascular Endothelial Function in Patients with Coronary Risk Factors." *Journal of the American College of Cardiology* 38, no. 4 (2001): 1083–88. https://doi.org /10.1016/s0735-1097(01)01467-x.

Johnstone, Daniel M., et al. "Turning On Lights to Stop Neurodegeneration: The Potential of Near Infrared Light Therapy in Alzheimer's and Parkinson's Disease." *Frontiers in Neuroscience* 9 (11, 2016): 500. https://doi.org/10.3389 /fnins.2015.00500.

Willis, Leslie H., et al. "Effects of Aerobic and/or Resistance Training on Body Mass and Fat Mass in Overweight or Obese Adults." *Journal of Applied Physiology* 113, no. 12 (2012): 1831–37. https://doi.org/10.1152/japplphysiol.01370.2011.

CHAPTER 9: HEALTHY LIVING— ANYWHERE, ANYTIME

Allahdadi, Kyan, et al. "Female Sexual Dysfunction: Therapeutic Options and Experimental Challenges." *Cardiovascular & Hematological Agents in Medicinal Chemistry* 7, no. 4 (01, 2009): 260–69. https://doi.org/10.2174/187152509789 541882.

Capaldi, Colin A., et al. "The Relationship between Nature Connectedness and Happiness: A Meta-Analysis." *Frontiers in Psychology* 5 (08, 2014): 976. https:// doi.org/10.3389/fpsyg.2014.00976.

Coon, J. Thompson, et al. "Does Participating in Physical Activity in Outdoor Natural Environments Have a Greater Effect on Physical and Mental Wellbeing than Physical Activity Indoors? A Systematic Review." *Environmental Science & Technology* 45, no. 5 (2011): 1761–72. https://doi.org/10.1021/es102947t.

Emmons, Robert A., and Michael E. McCullough. "Counting Blessings versus Burdens: An Experimental Investigation of Gratitude and Subjective Well-being in Daily Life." *Journal of Personality and Social Psychology* 84, no. 2 (2003): 377–89. https://doi.org/10.1037/0022-3514.84.2.377.

Field, Tiffany, et al. "Lower Back Pain and Sleep Disturbance Are Reduced Following Massage Therapy." *Journal of Bodywork and Movement Therapies* 11, no. 2 (2007): 141–45. https://doi.org/10.1016/j.jbmt.2006.03.001.

Fuller, Caitlyn, et al. "Bedtime Use of Technology and Associated Sleep Problems in Children." *Global Pediatric Health* 4 (2017). https://doi.org/10.1177/2333794x17736972.

Ganz, P. A., and G. A. Greendale. "Female Sexual Desire—Beyond Testosterone." *JNCI: Journal of the National Cancer Institute* 99, no. 9 (2007): 659–61. https://doi.org/10.1093/jnci/djk175.

Hamblin, Michael R. "Shining Light on the Head: Photobiomodulation for Brain Disorders." *BBA Clinical* 6 (2016): 113–24. https://doi.org/10.1016/j.bbacli.2016.09.002.

Harvard Health Publishing. "Relaxation Techniques: Breath Control Helps Quell Errant Stress Response." *Harvard Health*. Published Jan. 2015, updated April 13, 2018.

Hill, Patrick L., et al. "Examining the Pathways between Gratitude and Self-Rated Physical Health across Adulthood." *Personality and Individual Differences* 54, no. 1 (2013): 92–96. https://doi.org/10.1016/j.paid.2012.08.011.

Jane, Sui-Whi, et al. "Effects of a Full-Body Massage on Pain Intensity, Anxiety, and Physiological Relaxation in Taiwanese Patients with Metastatic Bone Pain: A Pilot Study." *Journal of Pain and Symptom Management* 37, no. 4 (2009): 754–63. https://doi.org/10.1016/j.jpainsymman.2008.04.021.

Khoury, Bassam, et al. "Mindfulness-Based Stress Reduction for Healthy Individuals: A Meta-analysis." *Journal of Psychosomatic Research* 78, no. 6 (2015): 519–28. https://doi.org/10.1016/j.jpsychores.2015.03.009.

Liao, Wen-Chun, et al. "Effect of a Warm Footbath before Bedtime on Body Temperature and Sleep in Older Adults with Good and Poor Sleep: An Experimental Crossover Trial." *International Journal of Nursing Studies* 50, no. 12 (2013): 1607–16. https://doi.org/10.1016/j.ijnurstu.2013.04.006.

McFadden, E., et al. "The Relationship between Obesity and Exposure to Light at Night: Cross-sectional Analyses of over 100,000 Women in the Breakthrough

Generations Study." *American Journal of Epidemiology* 180, no. 3 (2014): 245–50. https://doi.org/10.1093/aje/kwu117.

Morita, E., et al. "Psychological Effects of Forest Environments on Healthy Adults: Shinrin-Yoku (Forest-Air Bathing, Walking) as a Possible Method of Stress Reduction." *Public Health* 121, no. 1 (2007): 54–63. https://doi.org /10.1016/j.puhe.2006.05.024.

Nair, Shwetha, et al. "Do Slumped and Upright Postures Affect Stress Responses? A Randomized Trial." *Health Psychology* 34, no. 6 (2015): 632–41. https://doi.org/10.1037/hea0000146.

Pearson, David G., and Tony Craig. "The Great Outdoors? Exploring the Mental Health Benefits of Natural Environments." *Frontiers in Psychology* 5 (2014): 1178. https://doi.org/10.3389/fpsyg.2014.01178.

Salmon, Peter. "Effects of Physical Exercise on Anxiety, Depression, and Sensitivity to Stress." *Clinical Psychology Review* 21, no. 1 (2001): 33–61. https://doi .org/10.1016/s0272-7358(99)00032-x.

Sung, Eun-Jung, and Yutaka Tochihara. "Effects of Bathing and Hot Footbath on Sleep in Winter." *Journal of Physiological Anthropology and Applied Human Science* 19, no. 1 (2000): 21–27. https://doi.org/10.2114/jpa.19.21.

UC Davis Health, and Department of Public Affairs and Marketing. *Gratitude Is Good Medicine.* Posted: Nov. 25, 2015.

Zimring, Craig, et al. "Influences of Building Design and Site Design on Physical Activity." *American Journal of Preventive Medicine* 28, no. 2 (2005): 186–93. https://doi.org/10.1016/j.amepre.2004.10.025.

CHAPTER 10: YOU'VE GOT QUESTIONS, I'VE GOT ANSWERS

Heilbronn, Leonie K., et al. "Alternate-Day Fasting in Nonobese Subjects: Effects on Body Weight, Body Composition, and Energy Metabolism." *The American Journal of Clinical Nutrition* 81, no. 1 (01, 2005): 69–73. https://doi.org /10.1093/ajcn/81.1.69.

Ho, K. Y., et al. "Fasting Enhances Growth Hormone Secretion and Amplifies the Complex Rhythms of Growth Hormone Secretion in Man." *Journal of Clinical Investigation* 81, no. 4 (01, 1988): 968–75. https://doi.org/10.1172 /jci113450.

Hoddy, Kristin K., et al. "Meal Timing during Alternate Day Fasting: Impact on Body Weight and Cardiovascular Disease Risk in Obese Adults." *Obesity* 22, no. 12 (2014): 2524-31. https://doi.org/10.1002/oby.20909.

Møller, Niels, and Helene Nørrelund. "The Role of Growth Hormone in the Regulation of Protein Metabolism with Particular Reference to Conditions of Fasting." *Hormone Research in Paediatrics* 59, no. 1 (2003): 62–68. https://doi.org/10.1159/000067827.

Nørrelund, Helene. "The Metabolic Role of Growth Hormone in Humans with Particular Reference to Fasting." *Growth Hormone & IGF Research* 15, no. 2 (2005): 95–122. https://doi.org/10.1016/j.ghir.2005.02.005.

Pan, An, and Frank B. Hu. "Effects of Carbohydrates on Satiety: Differences between Liquid and Solid Food." *Current Opinion in Clinical Nutrition and Metabolic Care* 14, no. 4 (2011): 385–90. https://doi:10.1097/MCO.0b013e328346df36.

Schusdziarra, Volker, et al. "Impact of Breakfast on Daily Energy Intake—an Analysis of Absolute versus Relative Breakfast Calories." *Nutrition Journal* 10, no. 5 (2011). https://doi.org/10.1186/1475-2891-10-5.

"Sugar-Sweetened Beverages, Genetic Risk, and Obesity." *New England Journal of Medicine* 368, no. 3 (2013): 285–87. https://doi.org/10.1056/nejmc1213563.

"Sugary Drinks." *The Nutrition Source*, March 15, 2018. www.hsph.harvard.edu/nutritionsource/healthy-drinks/sugary-drinks/.

Van Proeyen, Karen, et al. "Training in the Fasted State Improves Glucose Tolerance during Fat-Rich Diet." *The Journal of Physiology* 588, no. 21 (2010): 4289–302. https://doi.org/10.1113/jphysiol.2010.196493.

Varady, Krista A. "Alternate Day Fasting: Effects on Body Weight and Chronic Disease Risk in Humans and Animals," in *Comparative Physiology of Fasting, Starvation, and Food Limitation*, ed. Marshall D. McCue. Springer, 2012, 395–408.

APPENDIX A: THE GROUNDBREAKING SCIENCE BEHIND CRUISE CONTROL

Amitani, Marie, et al. "The Role of Leptin in the Control of Insulin-Glucose Axis." *Frontiers in Neuroscience* 7 (2013). https://doi.org/10.3389/fnins.2013.00051.

Anson, R. M., et al. "Intermittent Fasting Dissociates Beneficial Effects of Dietary Restriction on Glucose Metabolism and Neuronal Resistance to Injury from Calorie Intake." *Proceedings of the National Academy of Sciences* 100, no. 10 (04, 2003): 6216–20. https://doi.org/10.1073/pnas.1035720100.

Assiotis, Aggelos, et al. "Pulsed Electromagnetic Fields for the Treatment of Tibial Delayed Unions and Nonunions: A Prospective Clinical Study and Review of the Literature." *Journal of Orthopaedic Surgery and Research* 7, no. 1 (2012): 24. https://doi.org/10.1186/1749-799x-7-24.

Brandhorst, Sebastian, et al. "A Periodic Diet That Mimics Fasting Promotes Multi-system Regeneration, Enhanced Cognitive Performance, and Health-span." *Cell Metabolism* 22, no. 1 (07, 2015): 86–99. https://doi.org/10.1016/j.cmet.2015.05.012.

Collier, R. "Intermittent Fasting: The Science of Going Without." *Canadian Medical Association Journal* 185, no. 9 (04, 2013). https://doi.org/10.1503/cmaj.109-4451.

Correia-Melo, Clara, et al. "Mitochondria Are Required for Pro-ageing Features of the Senescent Phenotype." *The EMBO Journal* 35, no. 7 (02, 2016): 724–42. https://doi.org/10.15252/embj.201592862.

Fayh, Ana Paula Trussardi, et al. "Impact of Weight Loss with or without Exercise on Abdominal Fat and Insulin Resistance in Obese Individuals: A Randomised Clinical Trial." *British Journal of Nutrition* 110, no. 3 (01, 2013): 486–92. https://doi.org/10.1017/s0007114512005442.

Fontana, Luigi, and Linda Partridge. "Promoting Health and Longevity through Diet: From Model Organisms to Humans." *Cell* 161, no. 1 (03, 2015): 106–18. https://doi.org/10.1016/j.cell.2015.02.020.

Gandy, Samuel. "Caloric Restriction Improves Memory in Elderly Humans." *F1000—Post-publication Peer Review of the Biomedical Literature* (02, 2009). https://doi.org/10.3410/f.1147350.604510.

Gioffre, Daryl. *Get Off Your Acid: 7 Steps in 7 Days to Lose Weight, Fight Inflammation, and Reclaim Your Health and Energy.* Da Capo, 2018.

Halagappa, Veerendra Kumar Madala, et al. "Intermittent Fasting and Caloric Restriction Ameliorate Age-Related Behavioral Deficits in the Triple-Transgenic Mouse Model of Alzheimer's Disease." *Neurobiology of Disease* 26, no. 1 (04, 2007): 212–20. https://doi.org/10.1016/j.nbd.2006.12.019.

Halberg, Nils, et al. "Effect of Intermittent Fasting and Refeeding on Insulin Action in Healthy Men." *Journal of Applied Physiology* 99, no. 6 (12, 2005): 2128–36. https://doi.org/10.1152/japplphysiol.00683.2005.

Hardy, Olga T., et al. "What Causes the Insulin Resistance Underlying Obesity?" *Current Opinion in Endocrinology & Diabetes and Obesity* 19, no. 2 (04, 2012): 81–87. https://doi.org/10.1097/med.0b013e3283514e13.

Harvie, M. N., et al. "The Effects of Intermittent or Continuous Energy Restriction on Weight Loss and Metabolic Disease Risk Markers: A Randomized Trial in Young Overweight Women." *International Journal of Obesity* 35, no. 5 (10, 2010): 714–27. https://doi.org/10.1038/ijo.2010.171.

Haufe, S., et al. "Long-Lasting Improvements in Liver Fat and Metabolism Despite Body Weight Regain after Dietary Weight Loss." *Diabetes Care* 36, no. 11 (08, 2013): 3786–92. https://doi.org/10.2337/dc13-0102.

Horne, Benjamin D., et al. "Usefulness of Routine Periodic Fasting to Lower Risk of Coronary Artery Disease in Patients Undergoing Coronary Angiography." *The American Journal of Cardiology* 102, no. 7 (10, 2008): 814–19. https://doi.org/10.1016/j.amjcard.2008.05.021.

Johnson, J. B., et al. "Pretreatment with Alternate Day Modified Fast Will Permit Higher Dose and Frequency of Cancer Chemotherapy and Better Cure Rates." *Medical Hypotheses* 72, no. 4 (04, 2009): 381–82. https://doi.org/10.1016/j.mehy.2008.07.064.

Katare, Rajesh G., et al. "Chronic Intermittent Fasting Improves the Survival following Large Myocardial Ischemia by Activation of BDNF/VEGF/PI3K Signaling Pathway." *Journal of Molecular and Cellular Cardiology* 46, no. 3 (03, 2009): 405–12. https://doi.org/10.1016/j.yjmcc.2008.10.027.

Klempel, Monica C., et al. "Alternate Day Fasting (ADF) with a High-Fat Diet Produces Similar Weight Loss and Cardio-protection as ADF with a Low-Fat Diet." *Metabolism* 62, no. 1 (01, 2013): 137–43. https://doi.org/10.1016/j.metabol.2012.07.002.

Kong, Ling Chun, et al. "Insulin Resistance and Inflammation Predict Kinetic Body Weight Changes in Response to Dietary Weight Loss and Maintenance in Overweight and Obese Subjects by Using a Bayesian Network Approach." *The American Journal of Clinical Nutrition* 98, no. 6 (10, 2013): 1385–94. https://doi.org/10.3945/ajcn.113.058099.

Li, Liaoliao, et al. "Chronic Intermittent Fasting Improves Cognitive Functions and Brain Structures in Mice." *PLoS ONE* 8, no. 6 (06, 2013): e66069. https://doi.org/10.1371/journal.pone.0066069.

Lu, Xin-Yun. "The Leptin Hypothesis of Depression: A Potential Link between Mood Disorders and Obesity?" *Current Opinion in Pharmacology* 7, no. 6 (12, 2007): 648–52. https://doi.org/10.1016/j.coph.2007.10.010.

Lu, Zhigang, et al. "Fasting Selectively Blocks Development of Acute Lymphoblastic Leukemia via Leptin-receptor Upregulation." *Nature Medicine* 23, no. 1 (12, 2016): 79–90. https://doi.org/10.1038/nm.4252.

Lustig, R. H., et al. "Obesity, Leptin Resistance and the Effects of Insulin Reduction." *International Journal of Obesity* 28, no. 10 (08, 2004): 1344–48. https://doi.org/10.1038/sj.ijo.0802753.

Mattson, M., and R. Wan. "Beneficial Effects of Intermittent Fasting and Caloric Restriction on the Cardiovascular and Cerebrovascular Systems." *The Journal of Nutritional Biochemistry* 16, no. 3 (03, 2005): 129–37. https://doi.org/10.1016/j.jnutbio.2004.12.007.

Patterson, Ruth E., and Dorothy D. Sears. "Metabolic Effects of Intermittent Fasting." *Annual Review of Nutrition* 37, no. 1 (08, 2017): 371–93. https://doi.org/10.1146/annurev-nutr-071816-064634.

Qatanani, M., and M. A. Lazar. "Mechanisms of Obesity-Associated Insulin Resistance: Many Choices on the Menu." *Genes & Development* 21, no. 12 (06, 2007): 1443–55. https://doi.org/10.1101/gad.1550907.

Smith, Ulf. "Abdominal Obesity: A Marker of Ectopic Fat Accumulation." *Journal of Clinical Investigation* 125, no. 5 (05, 2015): 1790–92. https://doi.org/10.1172/jci81507.

Stote, Kim S., et al. "A Controlled Trial of Reduced Meal Frequency without Caloric Restriction in Healthy, Normal-Weight, Middle-aged Adults." *The American Journal of Clinical Nutrition* 85, no. 4 (04, 2007): 981–88. https://doi.org/10.1093/ajcn/85.4.981.

Straznicky, N. E., et al. "The Effects of Dietary Weight Loss with or without Exercise Training on Liver Enzymes in Obese Metabolic Syndrome Subjects." *Diabetes, Obesity and Metabolism* 14, no. 2 (11, 2011): 139–48. https://doi.org/10.1111/j.1463-1326.2011.01497.x.

Sutton, Elizabeth F., et al. "Early Time-Restricted Feeding Improves Insulin Sensitivity, Blood Pressure, and Oxidative Stress Even without Weight Loss in Men with Prediabetes." *Cell Metabolism* 27, no. 6 (06, 2018): 1212–21. https://doi.org/10.1016/j.cmet.2018.04.010.

Thomas, Alex W., et al. "A Randomized, Double-Blind, Placebo-Controlled Clinical Trial Using a Low-Frequency Magnetic Field in the Treatment of Musculoskeletal Chronic Pain." *Pain Research and Management* 12, no. 4 (2007): 249–58. https://doi.org/10.1155/2007/626072.

Trepanowski, John F., et al. "Impact of Caloric and Dietary Restriction Regimens on Markers of Health and Longevity in Humans and Animals: A Summary of Available Findings." *Nutrition Journal* 10, no. 1 (10, 2011). https://doi .org/10.1186/1475-2891-10-107.

Varady, K. A., et al. "Modified Alternate-Day Fasting Regimens Reduce Cell Proliferation Rates to a Similar Extent as Daily Calorie Restriction in Mice." *The FASEB Journal* 22, no. 6 (06, 2008): 2090–96. https://doi.org/10.1096/fj.07 -098178.

Varady, Krista A., and Marc K. Hellerstein. "Alternate-Day Fasting and Chronic Disease Prevention: A Review of Human and Animal Trials." *The American Journal of Clinical Nutrition* 86, no. 1 (07, 2007): 7–13. https://doi.org/10.1093 /ajcn/86.1.7.

Weir, Heather J., et al. "Dietary Restriction and AMPK Increase Lifespan via Mitochondrial Network and Peroxisome Remodeling." *Cell Metabolism* 26, no. 6 (12, 2017): 884-896.e5. https://doi.org/10.1016/j.cmet.2017.09.024.

Whittel, Naomi. *Glow15: A Science-Based Plan to Lose Weight, Rejuvenate Your Skin, and Invigorate Your Life.* Houghton Mifflin Harcourt, 2018.

Witte, A. V., et al. "Caloric Restriction Improves Memory in Elderly Humans." *Proceedings of the National Academy of Sciences* 106, no. 4 (01, 2009): 1255–60. https://doi.org/10.1073/pnas.0808587106.

INDEX

YOUR MOST EXCLUSIVE OPPORTUNITY WITH ME

As a reader of my book I'd like to personally invite you to join my Cruise Control Platinum program that gives you the most exclusive access to me to help you elevate your nutrition, fitness, recovery, and mindset. One of the things I love about my work with celebrities—from Steve Harvey to Brooke Burke—is that I'm able to have a real, intimate relationship with their health. What was once available only to five or six people is now available to you. As part of your premium membership, you'll receive customized meal planners and shopping lists as well as live weekly workouts with me. Each day you will have the opportunity to ask any questions you have and get answers live. Best of all, you'll be able to attend three events with me in person, shoulder to shoulder. The spaces are limited, so make sure to sign up! Learn more at platinum.jorgecruise.com.

About the Author

Jorge Cruise is the #1 *New York Times* bestselling author of more than thirty titles with more than eight million books in print, including *8 Minutes in the Morning, The Belly Fat Cure,* and *The 100.* Internationally recognized as a leading fitness trainer, Cruise has transformed the lives of millions of people, including Angelina Jolie, Jennifer Lopez, Khloe Kardashian, Steve Harvey, Miley Cyrus, Tyra Banks, 50 Cent, and Eva Longoria. A graduate of the University of California, San Diego, Cruise also has training certificates from the Cooper Institute for Aerobics Research, the American College of Sports Medicine (ACSM), and the American Council on Exercise (ACE). A frequent contributor to *The Steve Harvey Show, The Dr. Oz Show, Extra, Good Morning America, Today, The Rachael Ray Show, HuffPost, First for Women, AARP Magazine,* and *The Costco Connection,* he also hosts The Jorge Cruise Show on Facebook Watch, as well as *The Cruise Control Podcast.* He lives in Malibu, California.

Automate your diet with my
nutrition products and supplements.
Train and transform your body with my fitness retreats.
Visit jorgecruise.com for more information.

---

jorgecruise.com
Facebook.com/jorgecruise
Twitter: @jorgecruise
Instagram: @jorgecruise